Historical Reflections on Care in the Western World

Beatrice Hale

Historical Reflections on Care in the Western World

Caring for the Elderly

palgrave
macmillan

Beatrice Hale
Dunedin, New Zealand

ISBN 978-3-031-87127-6 ISBN 978-3-031-87128-3 (eBook)
https://doi.org/10.1007/978-3-031-87128-3

This Palgrave Macmillan imprint is published by the registered company Springer Nature Switzerland AG
The registered company address is: Gewerbestrasse 11, 6330 Cham, Switzerland

Preface

This book is about care of older people at home from the past to the present. The societies considered here are Western or Westernised societies, reflecting my belief that this is only a first step in a much larger journey. And the care extends beyond the intimacies of care for the mind and body at home, to cultural beliefs and consequent organisation for the safety of elderly individuals at home.

While the role of caregiving is firmly established in contemporary times, I want to carve out and express its presence in the past by identifying different aspects of care at home, in particular, bodily care, including prosthetics, and also the more visible aspects of the spiritual and legal, of parish care, of neighbourliness, for example. I hope that some of this will provide caregivers with a sense of belonging to the significant role of caregiver.

The sources for my enquiry are as interesting as the results: finding, choosing, and reading them. More references and further suggestions appear regularly, adding or challenging existing knowledge. But there is always much more we need to know. This book can only provide the first steps to such knowledge, as I want to emphasise again. I have focused on mostly Western culture, but there is much more to be found in indigenous, Asian, South American, and African cultures. Well worth a good look.

To provide a context for ageing here, there are multiple sources such as spiritual, financial, and legal. And to highlight individual, personal experiences, I have gleaned information and taken 'soundings' from different diaries, memoirs, reports, and various other records collated by several researchers.

Though there is increasing historical research into topics such as gendered bodies, general medicine, growth of women's medicine and healing, the focus here continues to be on care.

Care at home for frail older people centres on the intimacies of bodywork and dealing with the confusions of dementing illnesses and cognitive impairments. In the past up until the later twentieth century, such a set of tasks have been tucked into the domestic role, hence making the work itself invisible as a specific role. And this domestic role was carried out by the women in the family, or by servants or slaves.

To begin the construction of caregiving as a specific role, I describe the work using information from a variety of sources. These sources include the spatial environment of care, the work of giving care, and interactions of the caregiver with others involved in the immediate care situation. These can be those such as home healers of herbal medicines, and also, at times, with healthcare and medical people. And the sources also help us build a wider picture of varying caregiver interactions, such as with neighbours and with close and distant kin.

At the same time, I want to note other systems involved with the elderly and their wishes, so I have included such formal aspects as spiritual, financial, and legal organisations, representing the cultural conceptions of ageing. And also of major interest are the social and religious organisations which offer general care for elderly people, from the apparently simple visiting sick elderly to the major social impact of health problems such as the plague, often leaving the elderly in dire situations at home and even in the streets too.

Carers and caregiving have always been with us, but much of the role has, as we will see, been contained within the domestic role, either of the women of the family, or of serfs and slaves working round the house. This invisibility, however, has recently been changed for a far more visible awareness of what this role entails. Public recognition in our times of the caregiving role has encouraged a sense of belonging to a particular group as well as ensuring a greater knowledge of the skills and knowledge of the caregiver.

My reasons for writing start with a personal interest and involvement in the work. Like many people, caregiving for me has been a lifelong set of experiences. As a teenager, I watched and assisted my family to care for my grandmother and great aunt at home. Later on, I tried to 'care at a distance' for my mother in Scotland, supporting my brother there who was the main caregiver. And when my husband's parents who lived near us became more frail, I assisted him in helping them. During those years, I never questioned the existence of caregiving. I took it for granted as something which we did automatically as part of family life.

A work of affection, yes, but also irritating and time-consuming. Disruptive, yes indeed! But present on the day, as a job, as part of the role of a family member, to be done because you cared. 'And you never know when you might need it too' was one constant refrain. Another refrain was 'Some day this might be you.' These philosophical statements urged on the caregiving and sometimes gave pause for thought.

But who does imagine their own end-of-life state? An imaginary state, with needs to be met, and possibly dependent on, for example, unborn, unknown children. So the statements tended to hang, as words in the air, pictures in the mind.

Subsequently, from the personal to work experience, as a medical social worker with older people, I found numerous caregivers keen to talk. And one particular caregiver suggested that a group of carers might be of value to each individual member. So with healthcare colleague Louise Croot, whose vision, interest and support was invaluable, we began Carers Otago, with the support of the late Professor John Campbell and the hospital geriatric units. Carers met as a group, fortnightly, talked and supported each other with sympathy and with practical suggestions. Carers were open with each other about their situations and, through their discussions, I gained a deeper understanding of what caregiving was about and the skills which care developed.

Without such care, what would have happened? Care by strangers in the home, perhaps, an increasing formalised service with the focus on remaining at home and employment of care workers. Likely there would be institutional care—a change of space from the familiar to the unfamiliar, and again, care by strangers. And institutional care is another story.

Care at home by family, as the group emphasised, is less visible than care in institutions with their paid caregiving staff. It is a more individual situation in private houses, and caregivers tend not to congregate much with others. They're busy, focused, can't leave the cared-for person and experience a certain isolation. But from those with their family members in hospital, and who attended the caregivers' group, I observed how much they shared and learned from each other, and how the sense of familiarity and of belonging encouraged them, and was for some, a real shot-in-the-arm. They were not alone in their experiences; from small to great. Eventually, we succeeded in extending the group to carers at home, who managed to leave their situations at times, here mainly on Western-based cultures, and I believe this is one step to a historical identification of informal care for older people. Care for elderly in other cultures, Asian, African, and also different Indigenous cultures, will, I am sure, require books of their own. But here I want to distinguish as far as possible the status and role of the informal caregiver, empowering this to stand beside other care roles. By highlighting caregiving as a specific role, my second major goal is to offer caregivers a sense of familiarity with each other across the centuries, and to generate a sense of belonging and a consciousness of being valued.

And so we begin the story.

Dunedin, New Zealand Beatrice Hale

Synopsis

WHO CARED? is intended to be an eclectic narrative of informal caregiving for older people at home in the community, an unfolding of different aspects of care documented by societies in the past, highlighting the often taken-for-granted activities of looking after those elderly in need. The societies considered here are western or westernised societies, reflecting my intention of making this the first step in a much larger journey.

Official documentation assembles certain aspects such as spiritual, financial and legal, which can offer ideas of the situation of ageing and the elderly in different societies. But to try and increase our picture of individual needs and care for them, I have gleaned information and taken 'soundings' from different memoirs, reports and various other records, to highlight often unexplored but essential aspects of care.

Of course before such care commences, we need to consider how ageing was perceived within different cultures, and how this might influence caregiving. And what did older people suffer, as, in our terms, cognitive as well as physical problems. But the main focus is that of care.

To emphasise my intentions, I will re-state that this is intended as a first step in exploring informal care in the past, care by untrained non-medical people, such as family members, household staff, servants, slaves, neighbours—anyone who accepts the tending, looking after, caregiving, on a daily, and even hourly basis, despite having various other duties in their lives. Generally speaking, such caregiving is undertaken by women;

it is a gendered role in the past, but men become more involved with care in our present times.

At the same time, there are other systems which include well-being and safety of elderly. These are the legal, financial, spiritual structures, sometimes called on to order, guide, and assist in care at home and in the community. And their existence and use reflect major social beliefs in the rights of the individual. So they need to be taken into consideration in our focus on ageing and care at home and in the community.

I begin with Neanderthal man, exciting work not only in its results, but in the vision which has brought this to our notice. Then I move on to early times of early societies, and their display of spirituality, and of abuse. From there, via early Judaeo-Christianity with its communal spirit of care, on to mediaeval parish neighbourhood help.

I've been unable to source personal feelings which are rarely discussed or made visible in these earlier societies, but sometimes I have succeeded in inferring these from legal cases. We need to move into later times to be able to source strong personal feelings. The strongest personal feelings on caregiving appear most vividly in diaries from seventeenth century onwards.

Moving into contemporary time I provide an overview of modern work, some of which describes the supportive interaction of individual members in small local groups. And to complete this work I outline the number of national and international organisations which have emerged, highlighting and supporting the work done by informal carers.

While the role of caregiving is firmly established in contemporary times, I want to carve out its place in the past, not only to demonstrate its existence as a specific role, but to provide caregivers with a sense of belonging to an important role.

And, as interesting as the results, are the sources for my enquiry, finding, choosing, reading, checking, comparing. There is much more we need to know. And this book can only provide the first steps to such knowledge. I have focused on mostly western culture, but there must be much more to be found in the Asian culture, South American, and African cultures. Well worth a good look!

Contents

1 **Finding the Threads of the Story** 1
Ageing and Care 5
And Onwards 7
References 9

2 **Soundings From the Earliest Times** 11
The First Story 12
The Second Story 14
Care Needs 15
Third Story 16
Care Needs 18
Fourth Story 19
The Old Man of Shanidar 19
Conclusions 20
References 23

3 **Soundings From the Oral Tradition: The Power of Stories and How Ageing Is Perceived** 25
Animal Fables 27
The Raven 28
Care Stories 32
References 35

4 Soundings from Ancient Egypt 37
Introduction 37
Sources 38
Carers? Why Not? 38
Who Were the Elderly? 41
Issues 43
Care—Where and Who? 45
Adoptionfictive Kin? 48
Care-Hands-on 49
Abuse? 51
Care-medical 52
Care-spirituality, Ma'at [Balance] 53
Conclusions 55
References 57

5 Soundings from Ancient Greece and Rome 61
Introduction 61
Context 62
Elderly 65
Issues 67
CARE-Who? 69
Fictive Kin 73
Bodily Care 74
Spatiality 76
Spirituality 78
Power 79
References 80

6 Soundings for Care By the Early Judeo-Christians 83
Ageing 85
Issues 87
Care 89
Care and Spatiality—Where 91
Care—Groups 94
Spoudaioi 4th–Seventh Centuries AD 95
Philoponoi—3–Fourth Centuries AD 96
Parabalani Third Century… 96
Almanah—Third Century 97
References 99

7 **Soundings from Later Middle Ages to the Renaissance—Fifteenth to Eighteenth Century** 103
Introduction 103
The Ageing Identity 103
Issues 105
Care—The Start 106
Legal and Financial Care 108
Kin and Community Care 111
Care By the Community 111
From Outside to Inside—HOME 114
Bodily Care and Orthotics 118
Noise 120
References 121

8 **Soundings from Eighteenth to Nineteenth Centuries** 125
Introduction 125
Ageing 127
Issues 128
Care: Kin 129
Care Itself 133
Place—Home and Community—and Movement 135
References 137

9 **America—Eighteenth and Nineteenth Centuries** 139
Introduction 139
Ageing at This Time 140
Issues of Ageing 141
Home Space 142
Formal Care? 144
Legalities 145
Personal 145
Gleanings? Soundings? 147
Sarah Gillespie—Her Turn 148
Conclusion 151
Part 2—Slaves 152
Stories 156
Conclusion 157
References 158

10 Sharing the Caregiving Experience: Soundings from the Media 161
Ageing: Adults and Care 163
Still Alice 167
Movies 169
Themes? Conclusions? 171
Conclusion 173
References 173

11 Identity and Voice 175
Bob and Eliza 177
Bill and Cathy 177
References 180

12 Modern Times 181
The Start 181
Colombia 186
Australia 187
Italy 188
UK 189
Scotland 189
New Zealand 190
International 191

Index 193

CHAPTER 1

Finding the Threads of the Story

Sources on ageing and caregiving for the elderly are multiple, varied, pertinent, inferential, visible, and observable, manifesting information. Some are peripheral to our purposes but still add to our knowledge.

Describing non-medical care in the west in the late twentieth and early twenty-first centuries shows us hands-on bodily care: cleansing, grooming, helping with mobility, assistance with medication and orthotics and prostheses, or apparatus such as respiratory machinery. And this takes place in the intimate settings of home, by bedsides, baths, often in the kitchen. Monica Green describes it well in her chapter in Ritchey (2021):

> The social organization of care labour has meant that status obligations as wife, mother, sister, daughter, and servant presume informal and naturalized obligations to meet dependency needs. Those needs are often accommodated in intimate settings, in homes and small communities, at bedsides, in kitchens and baths. (p. 260)

And such intimate settings tend to conceal any or all care activities, making them invisible or taken for granted as much as domestic activities.

A description of the activities of care often includes how the carer feels herself (and it usually is a woman) or himself. 'Burden' is one term that has been used. Steven Zarit and colleagues in 1980 and later in 2004, discussed the description of care, creating an index of the burden of care, an assessment list for carers to identify their own stresses. And in his later

B. Hale, *Historical Reflections on Care in the Western World*,
https://doi.org/10.1007/978-3-031-87128-3_1

work, Zarit (2004) discusses this further, focusing more on end-of-life care, and adding a discussion on long-term caregiving for the elderly, one focus being that of caring for Alzheimer's patients. In this highly sensitive article, he talks of the negative effects on the caregiver from the work of caregiving, on their emotional stresses and also of the immensity of the work and the learning which caregivers must do.

There are, however, positive and uplifting sides to caregiving. Two major groups articulating such positive feelings are some who care for Alzheimer's patients and for stroke patients (Mackenzie and Greenwood 2012). And the phrase 'labour of love' often appears in studies, suggesting a combination of both burden and upliftment, and introducing the idea of spirituality.

One question to be asked though, is what are the experiences of caregiving, the physicality, the emotions? Are they the same for everyone? What about the needs of the caregivers themselves, the individuals now more widely visible than before, it seems.

In the interests of this wider visibility I started looking round. My interest was caught by a fascinating book, *Prehistory and Compassion*, the work of paleo-archaeologist, Penny Spikins and her colleagues (2010). I loved it at first sight. It opened up more prospects and in more distant horizons than I had ever imagined. And it made me wonder what else had happened with care and the carer in the past.

So from there I began to try and carve out the role of care in history, and ask questions. What care there would have been in past times, who cared for people with disabilities, where were they cared for? And how did it happen? Were the stories we heard only myths? Did the ancient Greeks really expose disabled infants on the hillsides? In other societies, were disabled older people moved out of their homes by their families to beg and exist somehow in the community? Did family members care for older people or did they end up in the workhouse because women had to work, or because they had no family? Did the Eskimos really put their elderly on to ice floes and leave them to perish?

Direct explorations brought some answers, and there were often indicators for further pathways to follow; circuitous, meandering highways and byways, with words, phrases, and ideas to be followed up. The trail started with books and academic papers, with old letters and diaries, in libraries and on the internet. Sometimes I found information through the archives where I found both official and personal documentation. Often I found fiction, and latterly, I discovered the topic in films, where the emphasis is usually on the sufferer—see the movie *Iris*, for example, a courageous work about the writer, Iris Murdoch, on her suffering from dementia. With the fictional and film sources, even when the focus is on the sufferer, the work of the carer can be seen, or, at the very least, can be inferred from the actions.

Once the idea of exploring informal caring and its past took a firm hold, I could perceive care or infer it from almost everywhere I went or from what I read. Such inferences came often from indiscernible ideas, not apparent to those not interested in the care topic. For example, in the Fitzwilliam Museum in Cambridge, UK, seeing the prosthesis of the mediaeval metal hand began a sequence of ideas and thoughts about those who assisted in teaching how to use it, and who helped fit the prosthesis to the arm. The object also brought with it a wonder and amazement at the knowledge and awareness of movement of the muscles. Beyond that, there is a continued amazement at the craftsmen of those times who created such a superb piece of work.

Still in this same museum but further back in time, is a case of Egyptian shabti, or 'answerers', small model figures who accompanied the dead to the underworld, to help them in the afterworld. The Kunsthistorisches Museum in Vienna also has a magnificent display of such shabti. Look out for these in other museums. Carers? Why not?

So—on to the past. Let time stand still while we dig and delve. Or, as Oliver Sacks suggest in 'Speed' (2016) for his bumblebees, we, in our place, can slow down motion to watch carers in different countries, in different times. Using our historical imagination and following the lead of John and Jean Camaroff (1992), can we also become cinematic, perhaps, visualising carers at work in different places, different times?

We can visualise carers steadying bowls of water on their heads when they finish bathing the older person. We can think of carers helping to position incontinence devices, and attach prosthetic limbs. We can imagine the cared-for person arguing the case for better care and demanding more. Think too of tired women writing to other family members for help, of carers pulling plants from the garden to make healing lotions, or ointments; lay churchmen and women praying with the elderly and disabled—the list could go on.

This narrative is intended as the first step on the journey of a thousand miles, a warming up of the soil to germinate more seeds for further expositions of the reality of family and others looking after the home-dwelling elderly with disabilities. And the narrative is derived from 'a series of spaced flashes' a phrase Vladimir Nabokov used for other memories in his autobiography *Speak, Memory* (1951).

> I see the awakening of consciousness as a series of spaced flashes, with the intervals between them gradually diminishing until bright blocks of perception are formed, affording memory and a slippery hold.

My 'spaced flashes' are taken from a background of rich and varied information, with some descriptions of ageing and different aspects of care from different vivid historical environments. To say the least, each chapter could become a book on its own; I want to emphasize again that this is a starting point only for further work. And I acknowledge any omissions and errors as part of the need to continue the explorations.

The story becomes a weft of various strands of disparate areas: body, space, commonplace routine, individuals, household, community, legality, and spirituality. And we have a veritable bricolage to consider, taken from a variety of different sources: written, pictorial, archaeological, observational (see Matt Rogers (2012) for an interestexposition of bricolage research).

The aim here is to combine the varied specific experiences to each other, and use this bricolage to construct the carer identity, a recognisable visible status with a role, a series of actions or, in modern terms, perhaps we could term it a 'job description', with its consequent emotions. Using the definition of 'identity', the carer will be able to recognise what she/he and others do and feel, and are. To put it anthropologically, we are looking at a role and status which will then be identifiable as carers to the occupants of this role and to other people.

Where possible, I want to begin to identify caregiving itself in the past as a social role and status in its own right. Informal care will differ from healing and from medical and nursing health care. The care I have witnessed and what I want to write about as much as possible is that of everyday bodily assistance, meeting immediate needs, foreseeing others, responding to questions and cries for help, and general attendance on the person in need. This is the care we can all perceive by standing beside the caregiver, observing home care. At the same time, there is a social recognition of care.

This highlighting of eldercare at home throughout the past is intended to emphasize an overall value for individual carers in their present role and bring, I hope, a familiarity, a recognition and understanding of care situations. Along with this recognition, perhaps the book will offer a sense of belonging to an identity of caregiver, with its status and role of a specific social dynamic.

At the same time, I suggest we move beyond the immediate primary role to look at a wider care environment. For the elderly to live at home comfortably and safely, we might become more aware of other systems involved with aspects of caring for the older person—spiritual, legal, and financial. So we are moving beyond the immediate primary role, and creating a wider care environment, some of which will involve the primary carer through recognition and interactions.

Thus, here we have a journey throughout history, towards the acknowledgement of caregiving as a role in modern times. And, as Appudurai (1996) says, 'All major social forces have precursors, precedents, analogy and sources in the past.' So 'just what we do' as carer Rev Mary Webster put it, (quoted by Tim Cook 2007) has its roots in the past. 'What we do' is very similar to what we have done. In the past, however, there seemed to be little interconnection between individual caregivers, or groups of caregivers unless we recognise the growth of friendly societies as informal carers. Today, however, there are considerable interconnections and recognition, both face to face, and through electronic media. This recognition and these interconnections can and do contribute to the concept of identity, and, to me, they also contribute to the ideas of familiarity and belonging.

The exploration itself is interesting; immersing ourselves in other eras, other cultures, other lives. Since there are very few, if any, sources, which shout out, 'Caregiving Here I am!' the finding and selection are important in the eventual analysis of caregiving, with its multiple aspects.

Ageing and Care

And since the focus here is care of older people, the first of these aspects is *ageing*, not in the sense of demography, of how many older men and women of what chronological age—but in the sense of meaning. What in fact do age and ageing mean? Exploring the various sources for information on ageing needs will depend on an open-mindedness and awareness of detail rather than an undeviating focus on the specifics of health and ageing itself. And like those for caregiving, such sources can be subdivided into several areas: DNA analyses, reports, written on various surfaces such as papyri; records written on paper for different groups; personal letters and diaries; newspapers; visual material such as paintings or movies; literature as in stories; academic works. In other words, as wide a range as can be encompassed should be used in examining the accessible and available information.

If care is mentioned, good! If not, we can at least infer from the sources on offer.

Though many elderly interact with their families, caring for grandchildren, for example, there are also many situations showing that older people will work less, work differently, take more time over activities, will likely for many, have less money and will become dependent on family, and/or the state in many cases. And many older people will develop various age-related health problems requiring care by others. They are, in fact, an economic element in society which needs to be considered seriously: lack of productivity, probable lack of money, a need for health care, and a need for financial help. The outcome of these aspects can be care and assistance, affection, but also the opposite, where some elderly might receive abuse and rejection.

At the same time, should we not consider caregivers to be an economic element in society? Their care is free, and therefore there is no need for the elderly or for the state to pay for care. Until recently, caregivers gave freely. Now, in many countries, there is a small financial acknowledgement.

The questions continue: how does any social environment react to ageing people in its midst? Disregard? Supportive? And how does caregiving affect the families who see frail old people, and support and care for them? Care, giving care, taking care is often within the domestic and home-making role of women, a nurturance usually of children and, otherwise, a general 'looking after'. But, in previous times, there has been some recognition in the community, expressed through parishes, of care as a specific role, authenticated either legally by contractual obligations, or sometimes by a parish payment to a friend or neighbour for care of an older person and care for the elderly disabled in the community. Surely this could be seen as the forerunner to home care?

Defining caregiving for the older person is to emphasize that, in general, care is for a once-independent person, with specific tasks which the cared-for are now unable to do for themselves. The tasks are multifarious and time-consuming, depending on the degree of ability of the cared-for. These tasks, already noted, include bathing, dressing, grooming, for example; toileting; medical care, with the skills which that implies; feeding; companionship. And so on. Many of these tasks are quick, inconspicuous, taken for granted, and most frequently tucked within the domestic and caring role of women and therefore unacknowledged as a specific role; medical and nursing care are separate, with trained personnel in visible roles.

Although these tasks and the status itself, along with caregiving for other age groups, are now at the forefront of political and social knowledge, for long enough most caregiving has been much less visible, so concentrated and attached to the cared-for as to prohibit the caregiver to undertake employment, or much socialising. Such invisibility can carry with it considerable loneliness and isolation, not to mention poverty, as Rev Mary Webster discovered in the late 1950s, when she gave up her work and salary to care for her parents (Tim Cook, 2007).

And Onwards

Caring is now much more visible in our times, but a mixture of contemporary knowledge with the historical could strengthen and enrich the construction of the role and provide a sense of belonging based on a knowledge of caregiving for older people, sharing such experiences across time. Such care is worth studying for its own sake to clarify and emphasize the role and in so doing, we are carving out the role of caregiver from the (usually) domestic role, intensifying its value by increasing its visibility. Awareness of what happened in bygone years might teach us that 'the good old days' were not always the golden light in the past, and that our struggles reflect those of others. A knowledge of the past can give a sense of connection, and increase our sense of belonging to something beyond our contemporary experiences. Is it too much to suggest that with such knowledge there is a deepening of our senses and awareness?

Some caregiving experiences must be left to the historical imagination, where the evidence is patchy. This supports the notion that caregiving has been an invisible role; that caregivers themselves are unacknowledged or, that their struggles have not been apparent, or have received only limited acknowledgement in reporting.

So here I suggest again this is only the first step towards identifying the role, and I suggest also that we see it as a 'carerscape', a landscape of care inhabited by aspects specific to caregiving, building the picture from 'soundings' in each era.

'Carerscape' incidentally, suggested itself to me when I was reading Appudurai (ibid.) and his modelling of ethnoscape. There are also links with Christine Milligan's (2010) caringscape, or landscapes of care, and Sophy Bowlby (2012) who conceptualizes time-space links in caring situations. And the work of Jaco Hoffman and his contributors intrigues me because it suggests creating a collage of different aspects from a global examination of caregiving, and giving a sense of wholeness to the identity. This work of Jaco Hoffman and Katrien Pype (2016) on ageing and space and the practice of care in sub-Saharan Africa, is a must-read and highly influential work.

To provide my own 'carerscape' that picture through time and space, I have tried to 'take soundings'—with thanks to Peregrine Horden (2000) for that idea—from different eras, and highlight what seems to me to be the most prominent feature of each era. Each of these highlighted features will illuminate part of caregiving and, taking them as a whole, will illustrate the role of carer, as we see it now. By carving out such details and weaving them into this specific role, we should gain further insights into and appreciation of caregiving, while at the same time, by ensuring its visibility, we are in fact emphasizing the work of informal care as a major social dynamic with considerable implications. Each era yields their most documented and therefore principal aspect on caregiving, and by collecting and linking these in the final chapter, we can produce a picture of the status and role of caregiving, at least for older people in Western society.

The journey will take us from Neanderthals through ancient societies to mediaeval and then colonial America, and on to our own times. Each society has something useful to add to the picture of caregiving. For example, we will find spirituality and balance, community work, the origin of the notion of 'friendly societies' and outreach beyond our own societies, to start us off. Then we find parish support for carers and those with disabilities, and on to the personal and emotional inter-relationship. And throughout the book I have indicated features which, when combined, help produce the picture of caregiving, or 'carerscape.' Beginning with Chapter 2 with its unwritten material, we can consider the inferences of care from the analyses of Neanderthal skeletons. Chapter 3 takes us from the unwritten to the oral tradition, focusing on myths and legends to show how societies perceived the elderly and might or might not care for them. Chapters 4 and 5 focus on Ancient Egypt, Greece and Rome, those societies in antiquity with their spiritual, legalistic, contractual, and familial care, while Chapter 6 concentrates on early Judaeo-Christianity and its spirituality, with care as an outreach, and introduces its fascinating community lay movements. From there, in Chapter 7 we visit mediaeval and Renaissance England showing the power of parish communities and the recognition of caregiving. The next historical selection is in Chapter 8, eighteenth-century data from England and Scotland. Then we have, in Chapter 9, nineteenth-century America where family diaries and letters describe in vivid detail what caregiving meant to them, and explore the caregiving issues experienced by the slave population. Caregiving is now more visible and Chapter 10 focuses on fiction, many stories from nineteenth century authors, with others bringing us into the twentieth and twenty-first centuries, with a recognition of caregiver recognition, such as trans caregiving, and carer allowances. Included too is a brief consideration of movies. Chapter 11 will wind up the concept of the carerscape, discuss the caregiving role itself, and consider its needs for recognition, with a general discussion on the work and the status and role of caregiving answering my question of whether there are enough similarities to have an identity of caregiving across the centuries. And while cited references are identified, there are also lists in various chapters of other books of further interest, which may not be cited but I have thought them worth including.

Contemporary recognition will be demonstrated in the final chapter, 12 listing a selection of the different carer organisations, national and international, and a selection of political acts.

I should emphasize again that I have deliberately focused on identifying caregivers for older people in Western culture since the early explorations suggested a wealth of material. There is more to be learned from other cultures, so at the same time, I am fully aware and emphasize again that this is only the first step in the journey, and that more exploration of caregiving can and needs to be done.

References

Appadurai, A. 1996. *Modernity at Large: Cultural Dimensions of Globalization*. University of Minnesota Press.

Bowlby, Sophy. 2012. Recognising Time-Space Dimensions of Care Caringscapes and Carescapes. *Environment and Planning* 44 (9): 2101–2118.

Comaroff, John, and Jean Comaroff. 1992. *Ethnography and the Historical Imagination*. Abingdon: Westview Press and Routledge.

Cook, Tim. 2007. *History of the Carers Movement in the UK*. London: Carers UK.

Green, Monica. 2021. Afterword. In *Acts of Care: Recovering Women in Mediaeval Health*, ed. S. Ritchey, 258–264. New York: Cornell University Press.

Hoffman, Jaco, and Katrien Pype. 2016. *Ageing and Space in Sub-Saharan Africa*. Bristol: Bristol University Press.

Horden, Peregrine, ed. 2000. *Music as Medicine: The History of Music Therapy Since Antiquity*. London: Ashgate.

Mackenzie, Ann, and Nan Greenwood. 2012. Positive Experiences of Caregiving in Stroke: A Systematic Review. *Disability and Rehabilitation* 4 (17): 1413–1422.

Milligan, Christine, and Janine Wiles. 2010. Landscapes of Care. *Progress in Human Geography* 34 (6): 736–754.

Nabokov, Vladimir. 1951. *Speak, Memory*. New York: Penguin Random House.

Rogers, Matt. 2012. Contextualizing the Practices of Bricolage Research. *The Qualitative Report* 17 (8): 3.

Sacks, Oliver. 2016. *Speed* in *The New Yorker 100*, August.

Spikins, P. A., H. E. Rutherford, and A. P. Needham. 2010. From Hominity to Humanity: Compassion from the Earliest Archaic to Modern Humans. *Time and Mind* 3 (3): 303–325.

Zarit, Steven H. 2004. Family Care and Burden at the End of Life. *CMAJ* 170 (12): 1811–1812.

Zarit, S. H., K. E. Reever, and J. Bach-Peterson. 1980. Relatives of the Impaired Elderly: Correlates of Feelings of Burden. *The Gerontologist* 20 (6): 649–655. https://doi.org/10.1093/geront/20.6.649.

CHAPTER 2

Soundings From the Earliest Times

Timeline—ca. 18,000–11,000 Before Present.
How far back can we go? Palaeontologists say, 'To the earliest times.'

Penny Spikins et al. (2018) in reviewing evidence on Neanderthal healthcare, using a bioarchaeology of care approach, have suggested that 'the time has come to accept Neanderthal healthcare as a compassionate and knowledgeable response to injury and illness.' (Abstract). But they are cautious in their suggestions. Along with palaeontologists Dettwyler (1991) and later, Thorpe (2016), they agree that the data is limited and limiting, since there is little skeletal evidence to consider.

Evidence which palaeontologists offer for health problems which would need care includes dental defects, noted at different periods of time, and joint disease which was noted for the first time in the Mesolithic period (8000–4000 BC). Such joint problems could well be a feature of the lifestyle of a hunter–gatherer, the climate, and also of the ageing process. Survival from the problems identifiable from the varied analyses, such as obvious pain, broken bones, and other diverse ailments, including pneumonia and malnourishment, suggest not only that care was required but also that care would have been given. 'To whom?' is one question I want to ask. Would care be given to everybody or only to the most useful members of the society, that is, the productive ones, the younger ones, and maybe not the older member?

B. Hale, *Historical Reflections on Care in the Western World*,
https://doi.org/10.1007/978-3-031-87128-3_2

We could be considering two different ideas here. The first is based on the evidence of survival, despite traumatic injuries and despite impairment. This reflects a caring motivation with, apparently, no judgement on the individual's value to the group. And the second is the possibility that care may exist only for potentially valuable members of the group, given the cost to the group of the time and energy of caregivers and perhaps also the number of potential caregivers.

While keeping these ideas in mind, I want to begin building the carerscape by quoting four stories. From younger to older skeletons, detailed archaeological work has identified the needs of these individuals in some detail and from Tilley and Cameron (2014) there is considerable speculation on the care which they required and possibly received. Lorna Tilley (2015), one of the major explorers of Neanderthal health care, offers impressive details of early needs and caregiving, saying that archaeology rarely provides us with a representative sample of a population and this is especially the case when working with remains from prehistoric sites. Any assessment of the burden of disease within a particular community will almost inevitably be broad-brush at best, even under the most favourable circumstances (pp. 114–15).

It can be seen from the stories chosen, that I have extended a consideration of care from older to younger people for whom there is more information. And I have chosen the stories to represent different issues of disability. I have selected these for the details of their problems and the care which would have been required, and also to recognise the breadth of care offered, inferring where possible, and questioning when inferences are not possible.

The First Story

The first story demonstrates a major caring situation, concerning a man from eleven thousand years ago, disabled from birth.

'Romito 2' was a severely deformed young man whose skeleton was excavated from the cave of Riparo del Romito in Calabria. His problems were many: he might not have been able to walk at all or to walk well. To keep up with the group, someone would have had to support him or he would have been carried. Other developmental delays would have been possibly in other movements, his language skills and possibly his cognitive abilities, according to Lorna Tilley and Tony Cameron (2014).

From the skeletal remains, his diagnosis was one of 'acromesomelic dysplasia', a disorder resulting in short stature. In other words, Romito 2 was a dwarf. This problem is generally recognized at birth, and though people with this disorder usually have normal intelligence and are free of serious medical problems, their height is severely restricted and, as has been said, there were likely developmental delays. (Apparently an adult height typically would have been 110–120 cm). Also his arm movements would have been compromised, with mobility at the elbows restricted. He was therefore a severely handicapped young man, unable to take part in the work of the hunters of his group, but possibly able to assist the women to some extent with their gathering.

Tilley and her colleagues suggest he would need an extension of normal nurturing practice to cope with developmental delays. Such nurturing would require continuing care and additional carer effort but might probably pose few challenges. The thought is that he must have received this type of nurturing because he lived until late adolescence.

The anthropologists infer from the information on the length of his life that his group could and did accept his differences, both in physical ability, possibly to fulfil some role within the group, and also in his appearance.

But how did care take place? The anthropologists suggest that despite the small numbers and the stress of living, the group itself was supportive. They infer this from the information suggesting that he lived longer than might have been thought possible. There was, then, not only recognition of the disabilities but also that the group considered how best to help him.

What would be needed? Good communication and cooperation among the group. Lorna Tilley and Marc Oxenham suggest that group members possessed considerable brainpower, or as they put it, the presence of intellectual flexibility and organisational skills. These would be necessary both to manage the demand of the group on scarce resources, and to manage the demands made by Romito 2, helping with mobility in various ways, feeding perhaps, maybe bodily needs such as toileting, bathing, and grooming. And of course communication would have to be adaptable for comprehension and cooperation, if, as was likely, there were developmental delays and cognitive impairment.

Alongside the practicalities of care and adaptation to environment, there is also the question of emotions. How did the group feel about Romito 2 and about helping him? Perhaps love in our terms did not exist but maybe we could at least infer a sense of compassion? My preference here is to invoke the historical imagination, and suggest that there must be some emotional reactions, of both warmth and its opposite. But scholars such as Katherine Dettwyler (1991) have warned us against inferring emotion in early times, and Charlotte Roberts (2016) notes it too in her foreword to the fascinating exploration of *Care in the Past*. Nick Thorpe, also in this work, presents an interesting discussion on the likelihood of care, and on the possibilities of abuse.And there is a discussion of this possible care; a form of 'would it, did it, could it' as opposed to, 'yes, we believe it happened'. I find Nick Thorpe's thorough dissection of the different states of belief very helpful. He spreads out the information and ideas, grouping them together to make a thoroughly convincing 'yes' support for care in prehistoric times. Moreover, further work from Tilley on the Index of Care shows how she demonstrates the possible existence of care, with comments on the detail of care dependent upon the nature of the disability, and including features of the life context in which the disability occurred as well as the characteristics of the individual care recipient.

Romito 2 was a young man, and the inferences are that practical care existed. Can I suggest that since it might exist for the younger, it may well exist for the older. This is of course by no means certain. Younger members of society may have certain elements of productivity, while older members may be unproductive or limited in actions, and in need of too much family support.

So we have to ask: what about the economics of care? Does productivity affect the giving of care? If someone is unproductive, will they still receive care? And will carers step aside from being economically productive members of their group in order to care?

We can add these questions into our carerscape as ones to be considered later. What we have here are details of the disability and significant inferences on support and practical help with the activities of daily living. And I have to ask: alongside this practical help, can we also infer the existence of emotional care, such as affection and compassion?

The Second Story

The second case study, called in the academic works Burial 9, is a young man of approximately 25 years old, who lived 4,000 BP (before present) in Neolithic Vietnam. The presenting problem was that of Klippel-Fell syndrome (KFS) which, at worst, can cause total paralysis and at best is a fusion of neckbones with a limited ability to move the neck.

The bioarcheologists found that K_F had, from the age of 15, suffered from paralysis of the lower body and partial paralysis of upper body. With this came bone atrophy with possible complications of respiratory and gastrointestinal dysfunction, kidney failure, and pressure sores. He would have been in considerable pain and it seems likely that he would have suffered from depression. There would possibly have been a host of other symptoms too. Those symptoms described had a major impact on K_F's functioning. He would have had little to no ability to manage the usual activities of daily living, such as hygiene, grooming, shelter, or to eat and drink without assistance. He could not manage environmental hazards, participate in economic activity such as hunting or gathering, and would have had very limited social participation.

Care Needs

In his younger years, up until 15 or thereabouts, K_F might have taken some part in group activities. But with the onset of paralysis, for K_F to survive into his third decade, according to Oxenham and Tilley (2009), care would have been essential. Specifically, says Tilley, he would have been unable to eat or drink, to hold a container at the right angle, even to eat the usual foods of the group, requiring soft foods which didn't require much chewing or had to be pounded for him to swallow, and to care for himself in terms of toileting or bathing, or even to move independently even over the shortest distance. He would have thus been unable to participate in any of the group activities, to contribute economically to a very basic economy. He would probably be able to communicate, and therefore take part in general discussions. Tilley suggests there was no reason to believe his communication skills were affected. The skills required to look after him would involve liquid intake of a good diet with laxative properties This would require some thought and discussion and while perhaps being done to keep K_F alive, might also have included some compassion and relationship with the young man, as well as group concerns to ensure his care.

His bed and bedding, whatever these might be, would most likely have to be off the ground, both for his movement off the bed to be helped to toilet, bathing, and for others to help him. While in bed he would require support for sitting. Certainly he would need shelter.

Obviously, such care would include the provision of food and water. There might have been a special diet. He would have needed help with shelter or had one made for him. Likewise, he would have needed someone to make a bed for him, to ensure what Tilley calls a hazard-free environment. As he got older, he would have needed help with eating/drinking and managing hygiene, such as removing bodily wastes, and bathing. Someone would need to keep a constant watch to monitor his health status. From our modern knowledge, K_F would have had to have some massage, manipulation, and repositioning to ensure evenness of pressure to prevent pressure sores In addition, he would have needed help with his depression, such help requiring social inclusion in the group, either with individual contact or some inclusion in group activity.

I like to picture K_F lying on some soft plant material near the communal fire, being fed pounded material, given something to drink, and watching as dancers circled the flames. Perhaps he joined in a Neanderthal-type song. Imagination at work here can provide a warm picture of inclusiveness, while at the same time our awareness of disabilities showed how impossible it would have been for K_F to participate.

But back to the data. The archaeologists found no evidence of pressure sores or bone fractures. This suggests that there was consistent skilled care. It looks like this care was successful for a number of years, in a subsistence economy. Perhaps the community cooperated and gained considerable experience in caregiving, gaining knowledge, skills and ingenuity, understanding, and flexibility of behaviours. And at the same time, there must have been considerable ability to organise carers to assist, as well as the group to continue.

However, this is speculation, perhaps something to be kept in mind.

Third Story

The third story which I've selected is of a female skeleton named 'homo ergaster' or 'working man'. Walker and Shipman (1996) referred to this woman as 1808, eighteen-oh-eight, which begins to personalise her. I confess to feeling a thrill in connecting between the twenty-first century and her time of living of 1.5 million years ago. Stretching across the centuries to find that we are in touch with one of the earliest of the hominids, who might have shared a link with *Homo erectus*, or maybe was ancestral to *erectus* or perhaps had a common ancestor. There's more than a tinge of awe and excitement in this encounter as there is too in the others.

She would most likely be astonished to know that twenty-first century writers are interested in her. This woman, age unknown, suffered from a diet-caused disease due to excessive intake of Vitamin A, possibly due to eating quantities of liver or bee larvae.

We, the curious ones, are thrown in at the deep end. Where did she live? Could she talk? What form of communication was there? Was this a tool-using group? Did they have fire? The context of her way of living with her group has to be identified before beginning the inferences on what was needed to survive.

Or, maybe, we can start with very basic assumptions that in order to live in any environment she would have needed help. To live where she did, in the African savannah, help would be related to the particular environment.

The African savannah, a grassy plain with trees, water, and good light, allows animals to graze. Perhaps not the most difficult environment in which to live these days, but what was it like 1.5 million years ago? A reading on the internet will provide us with some information: grassy with trees, open habitat with good shade. The most common definition is a fairly open, grassy environment with a lot of scattered trees—a grassland or wooded grassland. Early man could wander at will, and be sure of comfortable shade if the sun was too strong.

Back to the physical issues. From the DNA analysis the archaeologists could identify a 'reduction in bone density and the development of coarse bone growths'.

Eighteen-oh-eight would have suffered from blurred vision, dizziness, headaches, lethargy, and lack of muscular coordination and impaired consciousness.

So what would happen? We can imagine from our own experience how movement might have been difficult, standing around a cooking pot could be tricky, standing or squatting to prepare food equally difficult. The archaeologists say that this woman would have had compromised mobility and presumably be unable to accompany her mates in food-gathering. She might be able to help with a little cooking preparation and maybe stirring the pot, but she might be severely limited in this and also she might be limited in taking care of her own hygiene, say, bathing and maybe even toileting herself.

She was certainly unable to be fully independent. But as a member of her community did she need to be fully independent? Or could she rely on assistance?

That's where it becomes interesting and relevant to this narrative.

To be able to identify such details in a skeleton, the disease must have been well advanced, and the woman old enough and having survived long enough for it to be identified from the analyses. As Spikins et al. (2018) say 'She survived long enough for the disease to be identifiable in her skeletal pathology, something which only occurs in the advanced stages of hypervitaminosis A.' Alan Walker and Pat Shipman (1996) suggest 'someone else took care of her', and David Cameron and Colin Groves (2004) say:

> 'There is no way she could have survived alone for long in the African savannah…someone must have been feeding her, protecting her from carnivores…. The group dynamics of early Homo must have been based on some form of mutual support. ' (p. 19)

We can begin to understand better what this woman would have faced and what her community would have had to cope with when we read the problems that others experienced at a different time. Alan Walker (ibid.) takes us to the difficulties which Antarctic travellers experienced with this hideous problem of excessive Vitamin A, saying that it helped him understand what 1808 suffered. He says (p. 134) from this contemporary knowledge the implication of care stared him in the face 'Alone, unable to move, delirious, in pain, 1808 wouldn't have lasted two days in the African bush, much less the length of time her skeleton told us she had lived.' He goes on to surmise that someone would have brought her food and water, having to carry both of these, with the implication of a strong receptacle Maybe that same someone or another protected her from predatory animals. Roaming hyenas, lions, and jackals were always on the prowl for a tasty morsel. He goes on to imagine that some concerned individual or individuals must have stayed with this woman during the long dark African nights.

Care Needs

The inference from the presenting data is that there must have been social care: someone to feed and give her water, toilet her; some to protect her, some to stay with her overnight, or keep her with them overnight. These all indicate strong lines of bonding and friendship, in our terms, and above all, care. Walker (ibid.) surmises that the protector could have been a relative of some kind because, as he describes, social groups among early hominids were likely to have been largely coincident with kinship groups.

He continues his discussion of care by widening the concept to mothers and babies, with primates, and on to elephants. 1808's mother would have probably been dead before the major onset of this illness so 1808 would not have experienced motherly type care for this.

So what we don't know is who looked after this woman, fed her, protected her? Was this a group activity? Did the care depend on who was best to undertake the specific tasks, such as protection, carrying water, feeding? Some care might have been left to older women, some to young men.

* * *

Another story will add to our knowledge.

Fourth Story

The Old Man of Shanidar

Next I offer information on the 'old man of Shanidar'. From the Smithsonian website comes the following information:

> 'One of the skeletons, excavated in Shanidar. Iraq, in 1957, is known simply as Shanidar 3. This male Neanderthal lived 35,000 to 45,000 years ago, was 40 to 50 years old and stood about 5-foot-6.'

The excavators found that this man was part of a stone tool-making group. Tools such as flakes, scrapers, and pointed tools were discovered in the burial cave. Possibly there were between ten and fifteen in the group, according to paleoarchaeologists, suggesting some form of kinship bond among them.

From Tilley and Cameron's Index of Care (2014), we have the presenting evidence for the Old Man of Shanidar to be multiple fractures across the body. The right side was the most badly affected; the right arm completely 'withered', with the forearm lost before death. He also suffered from degenerative deformities in both legs which were likely to have caused him a painful limp. In addition, he had suffered a 'crushing' injury to his cranium, possibly causing blindness in his left eye due to the deformity of the skull. Some archaeologists say there might even have been some brain damage as a result.

When these injuries occurred is not known, but it is thought they could have occurred in adolescence, but were largely healed with little sign of infection by the time of his death 20–35 years later than the infliction of his injuries. This is a point to be noted. His age at death was an estimated 40–50 years old, old for a Neanderthal, and equivalent to 80 years old in our terms.

Left to himself he would presumably have died from his injuries, but from the state of the skeleton it appears that he was undoubtedly looked after. As Erik Trinkaus, quoted in *The Source, WashU* (2017) has said, that Shanidar 1, 'like other Neanderthals noted for surviving their injuries and limited use of arms, he would have required significant social support to continue living until an older age'.And given that he was 'elderly in Neanderthal terms', as the anthropologists have indicated, we could infer that being 'elderly' was not to be dismissed but was a sufficiently important category for elderly to be kept alive. It is possible he was looked after by several different people, or perhaps a shared commitment to 'care' from the whole group. Older 'carers' might have died, younger ones might be busily productive in hunting and gathering, so perhaps some form of early roster could have been made up? Members of the group, suggests Spikins, 'must not only have felt compassion for his vulnerability, but also been able to talk about how they felt, and how to plan for his care… and he appears to have been carefully buried which suggests some form of affection or value.

Conclusions

Apart from the intrinsic fascination of the early humans, these stories stimulate a variety of questions and ideas on care. Questions are on the 'who' and 'how' of care, and the belief system which supported it. How were decisions taken, and who was involved? Given that the group economies required every member to be as productive as possible, it suggests from our point of view that different options had to be considered regarding care. To be weighed in the balance were the different domains of spatial, temporal and economic:

- The spatial-Neanderthal was a hunter–gatherer society. How could any disabled member keep up with the group?
- How then was the disability to be housed?
- Thoughts on the economy and what effort was needed from each group member; how was care to be given; how much time could be given up to care and by how many people?
- Temporal: how long might care have to continue?

How much time would be given up to hunting and gathering and would caregiving, therefore, have an impact on the group's economy? Virginia Smith (2007) talks of about three hours per person per day for hunting and gathering. That sounds as if there would be sufficient time for care to be given.

By exploring these disability and care situations, such an exploration does start our thinking on how care was given. We know that people were not abandoned. That clearly doesn't mean there was no abandonment at all. But it does mean that we can infer the early workings of care for some and we can ask perhaps who might have been preferred in terms of giving care, if indeed there was a hierarchy of caregivers and caregiving decisions.

Clearly caregiving involves multiple decision domains, and researcher Lorna Tilley in her several works discusses the complexity of caregiving in prehistory in considerable detail.

First of all, we can think of the spatial environment, and, as well as seating and bedding, we can consider certain sensory elements. Noise for example, and odours. If the disability and its care led to considerable noise, would this affect the others in the group? Would particular odours indicate a need for help?

The specific living environment is another: could he/she be incorporated into the main dwellings and share a hearth? Or were there peripheral dwellings for them in the different settlements? What was the environment for the disabled person and his/her caregiver(s)? Were there separate sleeping and living areas for those with disabilities and their carers? Were they situated in particular dwellings? Were the sleeping arrangements communal or separate?

Mobility is a third: Could the person with disabilities be taken out and about with the group, moved from campsite to campsite?

Another decision domain is time. In terms of time, what did caregiving mean? Were there physical and economic consequences for carers who had to spend lengthy periods of time caring? Were there considerations for length of time in caring, for time-appropriate care for each caregiver, so that there was a roster? Was there a time span for allowing caregiving to continue? For example, were people cared for until they died? Or were they abandoned, as apparently happened in later societies, when families were unable to cope either physically or economically.

Then, to add to our carerscape, we have the question of who cared? Individuals, the group, close kin, however they were recognised, group members, men, or women? What support was given to them as carers? Can we infer a form of organised care, as in a community initiative? Was there a family-type situation? Furthermore, could this be a community venture, or did some of the community become carers, while others supported them, all of them perhaps struggling with scarce resources. And could we infer any compassion and affection?

Considerable in-depth and valuable discussion of these questions for prehistory is undertaken by the aforementioned Lorna Tilley and her contributors, (2017). Philosopher David Doat in this volume, is shown as making ' transparent the assumptions, values and beliefs that underlie past objections to the archaeological inference of care, then subjects the bioarchaeology of care methodology to the same systematic scrutiny to test the resilience of the principles on which it is based. The author argues that (bio)archaeologists have a moral duty to provide an account of the past that offers a more balanced representation of our ancestors, pointing out that those with disabilities are often written out of the (pre)historic record, and certain 'softer' behaviours, such as caregiving, are overlooked. At the same time, he asserts that it is archaeologists' moral responsibility to ensure this account is as accurate as possible' (p. 17).

Most of the chapters in the current volume adopt a similar perspective (of analysis of care). They express the willingness of a new generation of researchers to go beyond, at a case study level, the existing pitfalls and past prejudicial scepticism in interpreting empirical evidence from the past.

Here, I think it is sufficient to say that while these questions cannot be answered for the earliest societies, the fact that we can look into these and use the questions to direct our ideas is important for further research into different times and cultures. And, as Lorna Tilley (2015) says in introducing the bioarchaeology of care approach:

> 'An instance of caregiving can be envisioned as a narrative with a beginning, which is the onset of the condition that elicits care, a middle, which comprises the activities that make up the care itself, and an end—the point

at which, for whatever reason, this care ceases. If an archaeological focus on care practice allows us to read just a portion of this narrative, then it may offer insights into past lifeways that are otherwise inaccessible. '(p. 12)

Further questions which arise are those closely related to the 'who' of caregiving in the temporality of need and care. Could the disabled individual contribute in any way to either the men or the women's productivity? Or did the needs require constant care from various women? What did it mean for the timing of camp moves, camp productivity?

There is, then, some concept of giving care, looking after, support or help, however we want to talk about it. So what else would be in this concept? Such questions and insights can begin the construction of a carerscape.

References

Cameron, David W., and Colin P. Groves. 2004. *Bones, Stones, and Molecules: "Out of Africa" and Human Origins*. Burlingon, Mass: Elsevier Academic Press.

Dettwyler, Katherine A. 1991. Can Paleopathology Provide Evidence for Compassion? *American Journal of Physical Anthropology* 84: 375–384 Am.

Doat, David 2017. What Ethical Considerations should inform Bioarcheology of Care Analysis? Ch.17 In *New Developments in the Bioarchaeology of Care,* ed. Tilley L, and A. Schrenk. Switzerland: Springer Nature.

Oxenham Marc and Lorna Tilley et al. 2009. Paralysis and Severe Disability Requiring Intensive Care. *Anthropological Science* 117 (2): 107–112.

Roberts, Charlotte. 2016. Foreword, Care in the Past ed. Powell et al.

Smith, Virginia. 2007. Clean, a History of Personal Hygiene and Purity. *Oxford University Press, USA Journal of Physical Anthropology* 75: 549–565.

Spikins, Penny, Andy Needham, Lorna Tilley and Gail Hitchens. 2018. Calculated or Caring? Neanderthal Healthcare in Social Context. *World Archaeology*, ISSN 1470–1375.

Thorpe, Nick. 2016. Ch.6, The Paleolithic Compassion Debate, Care in the Past, ed. Powell, Lindsay, William Southwell-Wright and Rebecca Gowland, Care in the Past, Archaeological and Interdisciplinary Perspectives, 2016, Oxbow Books, Oxford.

Tilley, Lorna and Marc Oxenham. 2011. Survival Against the Odds: Modelling the Social Implications of Care Provision to Seriously Disabled Individuals. *International Journal of Paleopatheology* 1 (12) (March): 35–42.

Tilley, Lorna, and Tony Cameron. 2014. Introducing the Index of Care. *International Journal of Paleopathology* 6: 5–9.

Tilley, Lorna. 2015. *Bioarchaeology of Care*. Switzerland: Springer.
Tilley, Lorna, and Alecia A. Schrenk, Eds. 2017. *New Developments in the Bioarchaeology of Care*. Switzerland: Springer Nature.
Trinkaus, Erik, Older Neanderthal Survived with a Little Help from His Friends, Quoted in Article by Gerry Everding, October 23, 2017, in The Source, Washington University, St Louis.
Walker, Alan, and Pat Shipman. 1996. *The Wisdom of Bones*. Random House, USA: Vintage.

CHAPTER 3

Soundings From the Oral Tradition: The Power of Stories and How Ageing Is Perceived

Even though we can't guesstimate the emotions involved with the care provided in those earliest times, the fact that there was care indicates that ageing and disabled members of the group were valued.

But later on we do not have to guess, since other societies have left more accessible information of how older people lived and how they were perceived, and cared for, giving us a general overview of perceptions of ageing and needs.

I suggest we do this by reading the variety of stories, sayings and proverbs, oral then written, written and pictorial in some cases if you want to look them up. Proverbs and folklore tales show us a way of thinking, patterns of information, and central beliefs, perceptions of elderly, perceptions by elderly. Some might be positive, with encouraging actions, some admonishing behaviour of the younger generation, while others might shock and horrify us to such an extent that the hearer/reader would be distanced from the story and its gruesome emotions.

For Neanderthal we would have to invent stories, as Jean Auel has done so effectively. But for later groups, we have a considerable number of stories. Many of these are folklore: stories from an oral tradition, now written down, teaching us then what to think of older people, how to think of them, and how to act towards them. How else did we learn then, how else create ideas, how else could we share knowledge? Stories are a most effective way of teaching.

B. Hale, *Historical Reflections on Care in the Western World*,
https://doi.org/10.1007/978-3-031-87128-3_3

Rather than following a timeline of stories, I want to pick and choose those which appear to me to make strong statements. What do they imply about ageing and the elderly and about adult children caring for parents? Look at some declarations. These are taken from Ashliman's (1997) collection on ageing and folklore, in which he quotes from Wander Deutsches Sprichworter-Lexikon, vol 1 But of course we might see them in any writings:

> Age before beauty.
> An old man can see backward better than a young one can see forward.
> If an old man lacks knowledge, at least he has experience.
> There is wisdom in age.
> Age deserves honor.
> He who does not honor age does not deserve age.
> It is good to grow old in a place where age is honored.
> Even bad parents deserve our thanks.
> With old men take counsel.
> Old men should be honored.
> An old man can be outrun but not outcounseled.

Now for other sayings, more focused on care, and these also come from Wander, Deutsches Sprichworter-Lexikon, vol 1, cols 54, 56, 58, 63, 1507:

i. One father can better nourish ten children than ten children can nourish one father.
ii. Parents love their children more than do children their parents.
iii. The old man saves, his son is a spendthrift.
iv. Good deeds are wasted on old men and on rogues.
v. Age pipes and youth dances.
vi. The parents' death is often the children's good fortune.
vii. If the mother looks after the child, both smile. If the child looks after the mother, both cry.

The first of the caregiving sayings suggests pessimism plus, as do Nos. 2 and 3. No. 4 sounds pessimistic too while Nos. 5 and 6 infers legalistic passing on of benefits. No. 7 is a deep one. Does this have within it the depths of caregiving: the grief, the emotions, the duty, the burdens of giving care?

Another general statement sets the scene for analytical interaction: 'I was where you are, and you'll be where I am.' This statement could be plaintive or defiant, depending on the context. It comes from the USC Digital Folklore Archives, and the contributor is an Italian-American student, who heard from her grandmother, who heard it from her grandmother.... and it seems, back into the mists of time, with each grandmother admonishing or reproaching a grandchild, or trying to induce sympathy and help.

When such declarations are handed down through the generations, it suggests that generational admonishment or inducement of sympathy is absorbed into a permanent cultural statement, with shades of meaning ranging from the personal and emotional to the relational. Personal could range from a 'look at me, frail sick old woman' to 'you should help because it might be your turn someday'. As well as suggesting that there is a 'duty' which the grandmother thought should be done, the assertion could be read in many different ways as the grandparent feeling challenged, dogmatic, perhaps powerful, or insecure, while the grandchild is focused on what s(h)e wants to do and keen to try something different or new, and perhaps contributing to the generational insecurity. The grandmother wants security, the grandchild may be ambitious and keen to be mobile. These selected proverbs or sayings on ageing and care have a variety of such meanings: positive and negative, warm and gruesome, unselfish and self-focused. There are ways of thinking suggested with patterns of information and emphases on central beliefs. And, like the sayings, stories, as we will see, can distance us from the actions of the elderly and potential caregivers, or they can draw us in. They can show us how people could think of ageing and caregiving, and what patterns have to be followed.

Animal Fables

Pessimistic views on parents and children and care are also reflected in animal fables. I've taken this example from Tolstoy (Fourth Reader, 1872). The first tale is mainly Eastern European and Yiddish folklore and I report these tales almost entirely, so we can get the full flavour.

The Raven

A raven was carrying his chicks, one at a time, from an island to the mainland. In mid flight he asked the first, "Who will carry me when I am old and can no longer fly?".

> "I will," answered the young raven, but the father did not believe him, and dropped him into the sea.
> The same question was put to the second chick. He too replied, "I will carry you when you are old," and the father also let him fall into the sea.
> The last chick received the same question, but he answered, "Father, you will have to fend for yourself when you are old, because by then I will have my own family to care for."
> "You speak the truth," said the father raven, and carried the chick to safety.

Father disbelieved the older two and believed the third. Why? Is it the young who count and come first?

> My next example comes from Gaster's (1915) Rumanian legends and tells *The Story of the Partridge and her Young* (p. 259). A partridge once built her nest in the furrows of a newly ploughed cornfield, and hatched her young when the stalks of the corn had grown tall and the corn began to ripen. There was food in plenty and safety enough for them to play and to frolic about without fear of any danger. But the good things in this world never stay long with us and this the partridge was soon to find out. The time came when the corn was cut and hunters appeared, followed by their dogs, whose barking they could hear drawing nearer and nearer. The partridge now began to be frightened for her young. She tried to cover them with her wings, but they could not help hearing the reports of the guns and the barking of the dogs. One day, not being able to stand the strain any longer, she remembered a place of safety which she had known in the cleft of a mountain beyond the seas. Tucking her eldest under her wing, she started one morning on her flight, intent on carrying it to the mountain beyond the sea. When she reached the border of the sea there stood a huge tree. Tired from her long flight, she settled on one of the branches of the tree overhanging the water. And she said to her young, "Little darling, see how great is the love of a mother and what trouble I am taking. Nay, I am putting my life in danger in order to save you."
> "Never mind, mother," replied the little one, "Wait till we grow up and then we will take care of you when you grow old and weak."
> When the partridge heard these words she tilted her wing and let the young bird fall into the water of the sea, where it was drowned. Distressed,

weary, and lost in thought, she returned to her nest and took the middle one of her three young, and, putting it on the wing, she started again on her flight to the mountain beyond the sea. On the way she again alighted on the tree with the branches overhanging the sea. And she spoke to this one in the same manner as she had spoken to the first. And he replied, "Do not worry, mother, when you get old we shall take care of you and show you our love."
The partridge, grieving at the words of this one, again dipped her wing and the young bird slid down into the bottom of the sea, where it was drowned. Almost broken hearted, not knowing any more what to do with herself, and heavy with sorrow and anxiety, her only hope being the youngest one, she returned to her nest, and, taking the youngest the mother's pet she tucked it under her wing and flew again to the mountain beyond the sea. Tired from her continual flight hither and thither, she again alighted on the tree with the branches overhanging these, and with her heart trembling within her for fear and love, she said to the youngest, "See, my beloved little pet, how much trouble mother is taking to save her dear little ones, how willingly I am suffering pain and fatigue; see how exhausted I am and wearied, but nothing is too much for a mother if only she knows that her young will be safe."
"Do not worry, mother dear, for we when we grow up will also take care of our young children with the same love and devotion."
At these words, the mother pressed the little one nearer to her heart, and, full of joy, carried him across the sea to a place of safety, for of all her children this alone had spoken the truth. And is it not so in the world?

So the ageing partridge does not expect to be cared for. But she is modelling the behaviour she wants her children to adopt.

To continue this discussion of the position of the elderly, we find stories of ritualistic killings in tales from the Brothers Grimm. No. 454 tells how in the eighth century, a community fleeing from enemy soldiers buried one of their old women alive to keep her from being taken captive. They carried out the fateful task while chanting "Creep under, creep under, the world is too sorrowful for you; you can no longer follow the commotion." This could be interpreted as care, or maybe the old woman was too much of a burden on the fleeing community.

There are two further instances of ritualistic killing of the aged offered by the Brothers Grimm and in each example the geronticide was accompanied by a ritualistic chant, which suggests that these had, to at least some extent, not only legitimized, but also formalized the killing of their aged (www.pitt.edu/-dash/aging).

But if we want to see the positives for older people, the Yiddish folktale of *A Fable of a Bird and Her Chicks,* reminds us to look up Leviticus 19:32, which tells us how to honour the aged.

And a further positive from Aesop (Weinrich, 2012), offers a different perspective in *The Old Hound*:

> A hound who had served his master well for years, and had run down many a quarry in his time, began to lose his strength and speed owing to age. One day, when out hunting, his master started a powerful wild boar and set the hound at him. The latter seized the beast by the ear, but his teeth were gone and he could not retain his hold; so the boar escaped. His master began to scold him severely, but the hound interrupted him with these words, "My will is as strong as ever, master, but my body is old and feeble. You ought to honor me for what I have been instead of abusing me for what I am."

Many stories show the practice of assisting someone older to die, reflecting the burden which ageing and care needs place on younger relatives. Economic burden, physical burden, safety of the young. …these are key thoughts in these stories of ageing and care.

Why? Because members need to be able to keep up with the group, take an active part in maintaining the group and not hold the group back. For example, in times of war, forced migration, or famine, the temptation to do away the weakest members of a group would be especially great. Jacqueline Simpson (1987, p. 40) describes a Norse saga of a famine in Iceland in the tenth century, circumstances in which, she says, loathsome things were eaten which should not be eaten, and some men had the old and helpless killed and thrown over the cliffs.

This resonates with other myths. Possibly the legends of the Inuit are the best known, where their elderly would be left on the ice to die. Such senicide was rare, apparently, except during famines, and according to Wendell Oswalt (1999), writing on the Inuit, the last recorded case was in 1939.

Another Inuit/Eskimo story sounds very matter-of-fact, again from Ashliman (1997) again quoting from Wander, Deutsches Sprichwörter-Lexikon, vol. 1, "One Winter there was an old woman who was left behind … with only a few insects to eat."

One ending is that she refused to eat the insects and for her kindness her youth was restored.

Similarly, and again from the University of Pittsburgh collection, a Chiricahua Indian myth tells how tribal members concluded that a certain old woman was 'good for nothing' and hence decided to abandon her. But there was some fighting spirit in the old woman. Alone, she wept to the Mountain Spirits, and they performed a ceremony that cured her of her ailments. She returned to her people and shared with them the healing ceremony, which became a part of their culture. The myth thus explains the origin of a certain healing ritual, but it does not directly critique the practice of abandoning an old, infirm tribal member to certain death.

And there's more! The following list confirms the negativity with which older, less productive, more needy people are perceived and treated.

The Heruli were a Germanic tribe during the Migration Period (circa 400–800 CE). Procopius states in his work, *History of The Wars*, that the Heruli placed the sick and elderly on a tall stack of wood and stabbed them to death before setting the pyre alight. For further reading, see Procopius, Book VI, Chapter XIV.

And although the book's focus is on Western culture, I can't resist this story from Japan. Ubasute is the mythical practice of senicide in Japan, and this apocryphal tale of the abandoning of an old woman is of an action allegedly performed in the past. An infirm or elderly relative was carried to a mountain, or some other remote, desolate place, and left there to die. For further information read *The Ballad of Narayama*, a 1956 novel by Shichirō Fukazawa, which became a 1958 film, and a 1983 film.

Moving now to Nordic folklore, the ättestupa is a cliff where elderly people were said to leap, or be thrown, to death. Apparently, there is no historical evidence for this practice, but the motif has survived as an urban legend, and is used as a metaphor for deficient welfare for the elderly.

Karl Haupt (1863), writing in the mid-nineteenth century, gives a particularly dramatic (and relatively recent) example of socially sanctioned European geronticide in Lausitz, a region in today's Southeast Germany. Himself a German, Haupt is quick to emphasize that Slavic groups living in this region practised this shameful custom. His account follows:

> During heathen times the Sorbian Wends of Lausitz practiced the shameful and gruesome custom of ridding themselves of their old people who were no longer able to contribute. A son would strike his own father dead when he became old and incompetent, or he would throw him into water, or he would push him over a high cliff (p. 9).

Indeed, there are many examples of this.

> Herr Levin von Schulenburg, a high official in Altmark, was travelling among the Wends in about 1580 when he saw an old man being led away by several people. 'Where are you going with the old man?'" he asked, and received the answer, 'To God!' They were going to sacrifice him to God, because he was no longer able to earn his own sustenance. When the official grasped what was happening, he forced them to turn the old man over to him. He took him home with him and hired him as a gatekeeper, a position that he held for twenty additional years. The source is from a folksong. And as a final survival of this gruesome custom, Haupt cites another Wendish ritualistic folk song, apparently still being sung as late as the mid-nineteenth century And then, we have:
> Old man, go to sleep!
> Young man, find a wife!
> Throw stones at the old man,
> And apples at the young ones;
> Old man, go to sleep! Young man, find a wife!

How far is folklore from the truth? Or does it epitomize the problems which younger people perceived in caring for the elderly such as the economic problems of feeding the family or group?

Despite what has been found in Neanderthal times, then, it seems from this list of stories that frail, unproductive older people are unwelcome in many societies.

Care Stories

However, abandoning this hapless, helpless miserable set of tales, we have some enlightenment through another set of stories. Care demands begin! We can see some form of reciprocity through another group of stories which show some justice and legality to helpless oldsters by awakening a sense of enlightened self-interest in the younger generation. The story, *Half a Blanket* is typical:

> A man had a father who had grown too old to do anything but eat and smoke, so the man decided to send him away with nothing but a blanket. "Just give him half a blanket," said the man's son from his cradle, "then I'll have half to give you when you grow old and I send you away." Upon

> hearing this, the man quickly reconsidered and allowed his old father to remain after all.

Could we consider this to be caring?

A variation on this story, again from the University of Pittsburgh collection, is a Hispanic version from the American Southwest, carrying the same message, adding the warning between the lines about giving a woman unbridled authority in household matters. The tale starts with the explanation that in the old days it was not unusual to find several generations living together in one home, then continues:

> A woman disliked her old father-in-law who lived with her family, and she insisted he be removed to a small room outside the house. One winter day the old man, who was suffering from hunger and cold, asked his grandson to bring him a blanket. The boy found a rug and asked his father to cut it in half for the grandfather. "Take the whole rug," the father said. "No," replied the boy. "I must save half for you for when you are as old as grandfather." The man quickly restored his old father to a warm room in the house, and from that time on he took care of his needs and visited him every day.

The story of the grandfather who is denied his customary place at the family table contains the same lesson of enlightened self-interest.

> An old man spilled his soup and let food dribble from his mouth, so his son made him sit behind the stove and eat from a wooden bowl. One day the man saw his own son, a boy of four, carving a piece of wood. "This is a bowl for you to eat from when you are old," he explained. He immediately restored the old grandfather to his former place at the table.

Similarly, from the Philippines is an unmissable tale:

> In olden times, when men lived to be two or three hundred years old, there dwelt a very poor family near a big forest. The household had but three members: a grandfather, a father, and a son. The grandfather was an old man of one hundred and twenty-five years. He was so old, that the help of his housemates was needed to feed him. Many a time, and especially after meals, he related to his son and his grandson his brave deeds while serving in the king's army, the responsible positions he filled after leaving a soldier's life; and he told entertaining stories of hundreds of years gone by.

The father was not satisfied with the arrangement, however, and planned to get rid of the old man.
One day he said to his son, "At present I am receiving a peso daily, but half of it is spent to feed your worthless grandfather. We do not get any real benefit from him. Tomorrow let us bind him and take him to the woods, and leave him there to die."
"Yes, father," said the boy.
When the morning came, they bound the old man and took him to the forest. On their way back home the boy said to his father, "Wait! I will go back and get the rope."
"What for?" asked his father, raising his voice.
"To have it ready when your turn comes," replied the boy, believing that to cast every old man into the forest was the usual custom.
"Ah! If that is likely to be the case with me, back we go and get your grandfather again."

So - caring is logical: you do it to him/her, and I'll do it to you. Or—you take care of him/her, and I'll take care of you.

In this set of mixed messages, where care comes from the grandchildren, and where care is expected to continue from parent to child, to grandchild, and elderly parent is ignored, it is clear that, somehow, care exists. Emphasis on caring for the second and third generations clarifies parental duties; emphasis on senicide and its reversion shows the force which stories will have on the morality of the hearers.

So, have we learned anything which builds up the identity of ageing and carers? For ageing, yes, in that wisdom is recognised, but so is frailty. For caring, yes, in the sense that caring is handed down to different generations, but is not necessarily expected from younger to older. But no, in the sense that the younger want to care for the elderly.

The significance is, I suggest, that the sayings and stories reflect the different aspects of ageing, and of caring, of the needs of the younger and productive members against those of the non-productive, of the knowledge of the elderly against the ignorance of the younger, of the will of the younger to care despite the feelings of generational continuity.

At the same time, does the message of the stories provide sanctions for similar behaviour in reality? They reflect custom and practice in some ways, but not necessarily the law. But laws are there for protection, as we will see.

The journey continues.

References

Ashliman, D.L. 1997–2013. From University of Pittsburgh's education/aging. And quoting Source: Wander, Deutsches Sprichwörter-Lexikon, vol. 1, cols. 54, 56, 58, 63, 1507. Sources: Wander, Deutsches Sprichwörter-Lexikon, vol. 1, cols. 55, 56, 62, 1507.

Astrov, Margot. 1962. *American Indian Prose and Poetry: The Winged Serpent Capricorn Books,* 211–212. New York.

Brothers Grimm, from University of Pittsburg website www.pitt.edu/-dash/aging.

Attestupa, r/AskHistoriansr/AskHistorians • 6y ago k0matose Ättestupa (ritual senicide)

Fukazawa, Shichiro. 1956. *The Ballad of Narayama May 1, 2008*. Proa Publications, Northern Marianas Press.

Gaster, Moses. 1915. *Rumanian Bird and Beast Stories*. London: Sidgwick Jackson.

Haupt, Karl. 1863. *Sagenbuch der Lausitz, Zweiter Theil*. Leipzig: Verlag von Wilhelm Engelmann.

Hoijer, Harry. 1938. *Chiricahua and Mescalero Apache Texts*, 33. Chicago: The University of Chicago Publications in Anthropology, Linguistic Series.

Jente, Richard. 2013. Proverbia Communia: A Fifteenth Century Collection of Dutch Proverbs Together with the Low German Version, nos. 181, 182, 525. Indiana University Publication, Folklore Series No. 4.

Griego y Maestas, J. and Anaya Rudolfo, Retold from "The Boy and His Grandfather," Cuentos: Tales from the Hispanic Southwest, 115–117. Type 980. Museum of New Mexico Press, Santa Fe.

Millman, Lawrence. 1987. *A Kayak Full of Ghosts: Eskimo Tales*, 184. Santa Barbara: Capra Press.

Oswalt, Wendell. 1999. *Eskimos and Explorers*, 2d ed. Lincoln and London: University of Nebraska Press.

Procopius History of the Wars, translated by H.B. Dewing. 1914. *Loeb Classical Library 48*. Harvard University Press, Cambridge, MA.

Simpson, Jacqueline. 1987. *Everyday Life in the Viking Age*. New York: Dorset Press.

Tolstoy, 4th reader. 1872. Fables for Children, Books for Children, ABC Books.

USC Digital Folklore Archives, http://folklore.usc.edu

University of Pittsburg, www.pitt.edu/-dash/aging Retold from The Old Grandfather and His Grandson (type 980, Grimm, no. 78). For additional tales of this type Old Grandfathers and Their Grandsons https://sites.pitt.edu/~dash/type0980.html.

Weinrich Beatrice. 2012. Yiddish Folktales No.12, https://aesopsfables.org/F231_The-Old-Hound.html, Shocken/Random House. N.Y.

CHAPTER 4

Soundings from Ancient Egypt

Introduction

The journey now takes us onwards to ancient Egypt, with its divisions into the old and new kingdoms, with brief forays into Babylon, Byzantium, and Mesopotamia. Our timeline is probably about 2600 BC to 146 BC when Greece conquered Egypt, and 40 BC when Rome conquered Egypt. There will, no doubt, be some differences in how each society perceived ageing and care but what I propose to do here is to consider in general ageing during this period, its issues and needs, and, as far as possible, the daily care given to people at home, with acknowledgement of societal differences and a nod in the direction of the formal healthcare systems.

To begin, I want to outline the various sources and discuss how we can read these. Remember that we are reading to find out about 'care', and remember too that in many sources 'care' as a definition is rarely used but, guided by our own ideas, it is possible to deduce its existence. The clearest sources are those of the legal and spiritual systems, where it is easy to see the focus on the well-being of the elderly, as it can be too in the general system of hands-on experiences such as pessary cups and prosthetics. But the emotions of caregiving are rarely, if ever, expressed in these earlier societies.

B. Hale, *Historical Reflections on Care in the Western World*,
https://doi.org/10.1007/978-3-031-87128-3_4

Sources

Among the most vivid and most attractive sources for ancient societies are the museums, either to visit in person or to manoeuvre a virtual visiting of the culture and time in question. Their displays allow for effective immersion into the cultures in question. The Sydney Australian Powerhouse Museum organized a fascinating exhibition in 2017, entitled "Exploring Ancient Lives", using the latest technology to go beyond the wrappings and discover what lies beneath. Another Egyptian collection is in the Nicholson Museum at the University of Sydney.

There, taking us back to early Egyptian society, are ideas of what happened to the mummified individuals. CT scans make the discoveries, something well worth watching on YouTube. Still on the internet, the British Museum shows its magnificent Egyptian displays and takes the viewer on tour. And in every Egyptian display there are the mummies, vivid representatives of this fascinating ancient society. Further YouTube displays will provide more visual information, with videos from, for example, *National Geographic*. When you are unable to make a physical journey, viewing, reading, and consulting the internet are very useful means for armchair travel.

But back to the museums. Something which caught my eye and has remained in my mind is the display in the Fitzwilliam Museum in Cambridge and the Kunsthistorisches in Vienna of those intriguing figures, the shabti, or 'answerers'. These tiny 'dolls', between 5 and 30 cm, accompanied the body into the afterlife, and were there to answer to requests and needs of that body. Each shabti had its job incised on its body.

Carers? Why Not?

The actual documentation of detail is as fascinating as the stories they told. There are recordings of early Egypt on petroglyphs, art incised or carved on rocks, usually carried out during rituals, and therefore with a spiritual meaning. Ostraca, these pieces of broken pottery with writing engraved on them, can be seen and studied too. Records were made on papyrus from the papyrus plant which was the major writing material for ancient Egypt until parchment appeared. Though weaker than parchment, papyrus was cheaper and much used.

And we have to ask: who were the writers writing for and why were various notes taken? One suggestion is that notes were taken for the legislature, as records to show engagement with the society's laws, and to be used in legal claims, for wills, for example. Some details in this legislation include cases of elderly abuse and these were used in cases of dispute over wills.

Some aspects of caregiving appear in various documents in legal, financial, medical, and spiritual systems. However, often the pragmatics and individualities of hands-on caregiving get lost among the generalised description of 'looking after the elderly' and we are left to infer ideas about such care. And, according to Sameh Elhabashy and Elshaimaa Abdelgawad (2019), there were female assistants or nurses but these were confined to wet-nursing, so were unlikely to assist the elderly, while doctors used male help in treatment and in medical care. So no doubt the elderly would likely have been cared for by slaves as part of their household duties, perhaps included with the care of children, as a general slave responsibility.

But to continue with documentation, I turn first to the medical documentation which might provide some information on care by telling us about the medical problems and illnesses of ancient Egypt with, hopefully, some indication of treatment.

The documents useful for our purpose are the magical-medical writings which give us some indication of medical problems and the treatments given. As the name implies, the treatments involve elements of religious incantations, and medications concocted from a variety of substances so noxious as to drive away the demons that the Egyptians believed had brought the illness to the sufferer. Treatment could involve the use of shamans to drive out the demons, but whether there was much influence on the pragmatic care to be given will require further investigation. Rita Lucarelli (2013) provides considerable information on the demons in various civilizations. She points out that people want a reason for the various diseases and physical sufferings. There are means to expel these problems, by magical spells and exorcism rites. With powerful spells to avoid the evil illness demons and of interest, she tells us that those health problems with no visible signs, such as headaches and epilepsy, were thought to be more demonized than visible wounds, such as poisonous bites by scorpions and snakes. There were other ways of dealing with these.

Alongside the illness information, we have details on treatment. If we want to know about prescriptions, we can consult the Ebers papyrus which contains details of illnesses and drugs, and offers 877 prescriptions as well as magical spells and formulae. The Edwin Smith papyrus is almost wholly surgical in character, and is the oldest surgical treatise on trauma. Not only that, but it takes a rational and scientific approach to medicine where medicine and magic do not conflict. This is likely related to the surgical focus of the papyrus, since magic is more likely related to the mysteries of internal ailments.

Details of other medical papyri can be found in a nicely documented list in Wikipedia with the papyri easily accessed. The Hearst Papyrus in California twentieth century BCE (before common era) the Berlin papyrus, and the London papyrus (nineteenth century BCE) are only three among others of major interest. Sources are scattered all over the world. And of interest to some of us, perhaps, is that the papyri in the National Library in Vienna contain the oldest known recipe for toothpaste a mixture of dried iris flower, salt, pepper, and mint. Iris is an effective agent against gum disease, and was much used by the Egyptians and Babylonians. Keeping the mouth sweet was very important, and toothbrushes, made from twigs with the ends frayed were much in use. So maybe it isn't care-giving as such, but that particular recipe could be considered as one of the tools of the trade. And there are others. Lucarelli (2011–2012) tells us to remember the incantations and the amulets, protections against malign gods and any demons of disease.

However, our main question remains unanswered: who actually cared? And maybe we need to ask exactly what care consisted of. Could we add magic to the mix? Since it was believed that many issues were the result of demon action, and magic spells were used to combat this, perhaps we could consider Egyptian care to include magic.

One excellent source for inferential ideas are the texts from the Deir el-Medina dig which cover 400 years of community living, and give not only medical but also social welfare information. Deir el-Medina dates from 1541 BCE and has numerous ostraca, detailing everyday lives in that desert region. Of particular interest here is a cult of domesticity describing the varied positions and work of women. There are references to the altars celebrating feminine deities, one of whom is Bastet, the goddess of hearth, home, women, children, and women's secrets. And we find too that there were people who had adult children and grandchildren. Definitely indicators of an ageing population.

Other sources include books, written teachings and demographic information and, importantly, "The Wisdom Texts", with their focus on spirituality and health and, to my mind, inferring a notion of self-care. All these are useful in our efforts at creating an idea of caregiving.

As well as the above, there are the texts for teaching, and cautionary tales reminding people how to lead a virtuous life. While there is no general literacy in ancient societies, those who could read such texts would be able to tell others how to live and behave. Another audience was the literate professional recipients of information able to read and understand a variety of texts, in particular, documents such as wills. Those which survive show the transmission of property, often in return for care, maybe the first glimmerings of caregiving.

Who Were the Elderly?

Who were the elderly? Most of the information is demographic. In the chronology of growing up and growing older, data show that there were many children who didn't reach adulthood, women often died in childbirth, and diseases, now treatable, were actually fatal for the ancient Egyptians. I wonder whether the mindset could have been one of expecting the worst, such as death and disability, rather than healing and curing and living, despite the optimism of the herbal and spiritual healing. Perhaps rather than expecting old age, men and women must have had to prepare themselves for the death of a wife or a child and then move on.

The demographic descriptions for those who did reach older ages is sometimes positive and sometimes negative. Although the early thirties have been suggested as 'old age' for Egyptians, by Winkler and Wilfling, who say also that 'old age' was perceived when the older adult was unable to contribute labour (from a blog post "On Ancient Egypt" by Ann Liljas in 2015). A Babylonian text lays down a very clear definition without adding detail of what each stage means. Quoted from Martha T. Roth, we find: 40 (years) is the prime of life, 50 is short life, 60 is maturity, 70 is longevity, 80 is grey hairs, 90 is extreme old age" (1987).

Thoth, a highly significant god in the Egyptian Pantheon, is more positive. He has assigned sixty years more of life to men and women, so from the age of 40 to the expected 100, a man could enjoy the best years of his life, using the results of his labour and knowledge. The Egyptians regarded the attainment of this age as evidence of special divine favour and the reward for blameless behaviour. And such old people therefore were respected for their experience and wisdom, and their wise advice received close attention.

Concluding these references to the numbers game, there is a list in Mishnaic Hebrew which laid down, inter alia: '…40 for discernment, 50 for counsel, 60 for old age, 70 for grey hairs, 80 for strength, 90 for bowed back, 100: as though he were dead and had passed away and ceased from the world' (Avot 5:21).

But the elderly were needed, as teaching from Ptahhotep, a vizier from the late twenty-fifth and early twenty-fourth centuries BC, is clear.

The king, who is old, is requested to retire and consents to this request but he also observes that the young need the old. according to Ptahotep, in his 'Maxims" 'none can be born wise'. A clear moral precept here for the children and grandchildren.

Ageing, as well as being related to figures, is perceived as a stage of reduced productivity. Men who were unable to complete their jobs and who had to quit these jobs could be considered old. Women's ageing was less obvious, since those who worked at home would be more or less invisible But in terms of ageing, women were described in terms of reproductive capacity, as well as their decreasing domestic work, and of course, their appearance, altered naturally by the ageing process. However, when women worked outside the home they could, like the men, be considered old when they were no longer able to work, or at least work as productively as they used to do. Activities which demanded considerable physical energy would diminish, while activities requiring knowledge and skills 'which improve with practice' would gain the older women more work, and more appreciation. Visible ageing and its concomitant issues gave rise to perceptions of the elderly in behavioural terms: wise, spiritual, and useful or spiteful, fearful, and ugly. Such descriptions and perceptions suggest that the body is an important defining element in ageing. The elderly body is perceived through its use or non-use, its decay, and its treatment as a biological or medical problem to be cured. Or cared for.

What then was the lived experience of ordinary older people, especially those in need of some help? Being avoided, or insulted, not working, probably poor, walking, shuffling, limping, having to be helped to get up and out, walking with a staff. And many other issues might be invisible. The obvious question, of course, is whether or how much physical appearance influences perceptions, behaviour, and treatment, and consequently caregiving.

Issues

What we need to know now is what are the problems afflicting older people which require care. These are identified in various papyri connected with ill health, such as arthritis, joint pain, paralysis, blindness, and deafness. Arthritis and dental problems are features of many ancient societies, and ancient Egypt was no exception. Although arthritis could set in after an accident or infection, generally it would be a consequence of the ageing process. It should be noted, though, that mummified remains came from the higher social classes (David et al. 2010) and there might have been more problems in the lower classes.

Atherosclerosis seems to have been especially prevalent among the upper classes and their families, most likely due to diets high in unsaturated fats, and the priests in particular had consumed their fill, according to a number of authors (Allam et al. 2014; David et al. ibid.) Other information shows evidence of serious conditions, such as tuberculosis, leprosy, tumours, and polio. And cleft palate has also been noted in exhumed Egyptian and Nubian bodies (africame.factsanddetails.com/article/entry-202.html-). Look for the section on Health of Ancient Egyptians as seen through their bones. Presumably these victims were nursed either at home or perhaps in the nearest temple of healing. And, as I have already noted in this chapter, there were magic spells against illness demons, and exorcism rites to expel demonized diseases from the body (Lucarelli 2013).

And whether we can refer to dental problems as a disability, or not, the information is interesting. We have some detailed dental information in the *British Dental Journal* (2009) in an article by Forshaw, where he says the most frequent pathological condition identified was that of excessive tooth wear, a condition so widespread that it was found in most of the ancient Egyptian skulls throughout the dynastic period.

F. Leek (1996) in a study of 4,800 ancient Egyptian teeth, found that nearly 90% of the teeth showed some evidence of tooth wear. This disorder has often been categorized as attrition, but analysis of the problem reveals that attrition was not the sole agent responsible for the loss of tooth tissue. There was also contamination of food, and of course, tooth wear increased with age.

Disability in general was given respect, ingrained into the 'wisdom teachings' of the culture. Dwarfism, for example, was held in high respect in ancient Egypt, and also ingrained into the 'wisdom teachings' of the culture with their principle focus of cultivating understanding, peace, harmony, selfless service, self-control, and inner fulfilment with spiritual realization. Amenemope, (dating within broad limits of 1000–600 BCE), a wise man who lived during the New Kingdom, wrote that care for the old, the sick, and the malformed was a moral duty. 'Man is clay and straw, the God is his builder,' Amenemope wrote in The Instruction of Amenemope, of moral teaching, discussed in worldhistoryedu.com. The Wise Man should respect people affected by reversal of fortune.

And despite the ingrained wisdom teachings, as regards the elderly in particular, we have the following, rather gloomy description: the teaching of the Overseer of the City and Vizier Ptahhotep before the power of the dual king Isesi living for ever and eternity. The Overseer of the City and Vizier Ptahhotep declares:

> O my sovereign,
> Old age has struck, age has descended,
> Feebleness has arrived, weakness is here again.
> Sleep is upon him in discomfort all day.
> Eyes are grown small, ears deaf,
> Mouth silent, unable to speak,
> Heart emptied, unable to recall yesterday.
> Bones ache his whole length.
> Goodness has turned to evil,
> All taste is gone.
> What old age does to people is evil in every way.
> Nose is blocked, unable to breathe,
> how old (it feels) standing or sitting.
> Let a staff of old age be decreed to be made for this humble servant.
> Let him be told the speech of those who assess,
> the advice of the ancestors once heard by the gods.
> Then the same may be done for you,
> strife may be removed from the populace,
> and the Two Shores may toil for you.

Just to add to the grim list above, there is mention of parasites, such as guinea worms.

So to caregiving—and the major questions therein: who looked after these people, what was the care and how was it managed?

Care—Where and Who?

If we walk through an Egyptian village in search for older people, we will be jostled and will jostle in our turn because these villages tend to be crowded. Living arrangements for the poorer Egyptians were that they often lived with their whole family in only one room of a mudbrick house, with more families living in the other rooms. This kind of apartment house involved other families as neighbours, not necessarily relatives. Historians such as Rosalind and Jac Janssen (1996), among others, who have looked at contracts and ancient tax records have shown that such a building was more like an apartment house, though all the families shared the use of the courtyard. There would always be someone around to help, so care would have been unavoidable in such a confined space. It was likely that there would be neighbourly help available if the families could not cope by themselves, or even for those living by themselves, should there be such.

As well as one-room homes in apartment buildings, there were also mud huts for the poorest and the Egyptian peasant occupied a small and squalid hut of mudbrick or clay-daubed reed matting. Ceilings were made from bundles of plant stems, and the floors consisted of hard-beaten earth covered with a layer of straw or reed mats. There were one or two rooms (perhaps occasionally three) in which the farmer and his wife and children (if any) lived. In many cases, they stabled some or all of their farm animals in the same rooms.

Bed and bedding would have taken up some space, either to remain if needed for sick people or to be removed to create some space for moving around, cooking, and eating.

Lying on the floor, with perhaps a mat underneath, the older person would have needed help to move around. Farmers' wives were involved in keeping the house clean, tending to any animals not used in ploughing, looking after the children and also taking care of the elderly in the family, though whether there was help from servants or slaves is not clear. There was no space for bathrooms or anything like a toilet, so the residents had to use an outside latrine, hole in the ground, to relieve themselves. And water for all purposes had to be hauled in buckets from the river or the nearest hand-dug well.

In these cramped quarters a household would include one's aged parents. An entry quoted by Marie Parsons, a https://www.touregypt.net/featurestories/oldage.htm

From the workmen's town of Kahun in ancient Egypt shows a household list which reads, somewhat confusingly:

> The soldier, Dhutis son Hori;
> His wife, Satsopdus daughter Shepset;
> Their son Snefru;
> Horis mother Harekni;
> Her daughters, Qatsennut, Mekten, Ese, Rudet, and Satsnefru.

Should Hori's mother require help, there would be plenty of people around. This might include slaves for some people, though there are none mentioned in Hori's household, but apparently slaves were less used in households than in other areas of work.

In terms of day-to-day hands-on care, the nuclear family was all-important for regular help and support. It was the core of Egyptian society. Children were morally obliged to care for their parents: the kin group had major responsibilities. From the work of Brewer and Teeter (2007) we hear that:

> The nuclear family was the core of Egyptian society and many of the gods were even arranged into such groupings. There was tremendous pride in one's family, and lineage was traced through both the mother's and father's lines. Respect for one's parents was a cornerstone of morality, and the most fundamental duty of the eldest son or daughter was to care for his/her parents in their last days and to ensure that they received a proper burial. (p. 1)

So kinship care seems to be taken for granted, wherever there were adult children. The type of care given would be a mixture of oversight and hands-on care. Supervision of financial, social, and spiritual needs could be done by sons or daughters, but it is likely that the hands-on care would be carried out by the women in the family, servants or possibly slaves.

Included in kinship care is undoubtedly the financing of the older people whether this is in actual money or in food. An ancient Egyptian pension scheme was where the worker donated to a god or goddess, usually Ma'at, and this might be added to by donations from other family members to ensure a pension in non-productive years.

As well as money, there was food to be provided. McDowell (1998), author of the pension information, says Weskmenhet gave his father half his monthly wage. He earned 5 and a half sacks of rations, but in the text it says,

> And I gave to bim emmer amounting to 2 ½ sacks as rations every month from year 1 until year 2, second month of the inundation season to third month of the summer season, making 0 months, each 2 ½ sacks. Total 27 ½ sacks. (p. 210)

Yet another form of ensuring a cash flow between generations is to enter into reciprocal arrangements with the adult child. The elderly give the adult child goods and the adult child returns the compliment with either money or food. One story suggests that:

The workman Khaemnun bequeathed a bronze washing-bowl weighing 13 debens of copper to his son Kenherkhepeshef on condition that the latter provide him with a monthly stipend.

Another reference says that Khaemnum bequeathed this to his wife. And there were similar arrangements for women, especially widowed and divorced women, but whether old or not is not clear, says 'McDowell in Stoll and Vleeming (1998, p. 213)'. This arrangement, as McDowell emphasies, was one of reciprocity, along the lines of you help me and I'll give you. She quotes the situation of Naumakhte who disinherited the children who hadn't helped her, and favoured those who had. But more on that situation later.

There was no possibility of individual choices of work. Herodotus and Diodorus both refer to a hereditary calling of sons following fathers, and rather than a system of rigid inheritance, this was more of an effort to pass on a father's functions to his children. Sons were described as 'the staff of his father's old age' and were to assist their fathers, and eventually succeed them This made it an automatic set of actions to care for father, and presumably mother too, when they became incapacitated. There was no other path to take.

And to emphasize it, there were instructions in literature on how to behave to ageing parents. These tales were sometimes autobiographical, and sometimes mythological and story-fashion.

Respect for one's parents was thus built into society in a number of ways: legally, socially, and morally. A veritable cornerstone of morality as *The Instruction of Ani* reminds us: 'Never remain seated if a man older than yourself is standing.' Ani appears to be a minor official in the New Kingdom and Eighteenth Dynasty, and writes instructively for the middle class or the ordinary person (see http://www.perankhgroup.com/index.htm for more of what Ani says).

Adoptionfictive Kin?

The thought of an old age without children's support was horrific. Something had to happen, both for care and for someone to leave the estate to, at least for the wealthy. Stol (1998) talks in terms of a contingency plan, that of adoption, quite common apparently, for childless couples. One New Kingdom ostracon (pottery used as notebook) relates, 'As for him who has no children, he adopts an orphan instead [to] bring him up' (https://fathom.lib.uchicago.edu/2/21701778/#). Other examples in this library are of a man who 'adopted' his brother and of a woman named Nau-nakht, who had other children, but who adopted and reared the freed children of her female servant because of the kindness that they showed to her.

It seems a complex business, involving legal transfer of kinship roles, an interesting and highly complex situation, according to pundits such as Rivkah Harris (1992).

Caring for the elderly in ancient societies is a fascinating mish-mash, it seems, of various contracts, of adoption, of rituals to ensure that adoptees and/or slaves were freed after their caring responsibilities were over.

Further information to be gleaned comes from an Old Babylonian text whereby two men were entrusted by a husband to support his wife for life, and in return, on his death they are his heirs. But fourteen years later on, one of them assigns a slave for her care in his stead. When she dies the slave returns to the man who assigned him. And presumably he was still an heir.

And more comments on adoption come from a neo-Babylonian text which discusses adoption of the wife's granddaughter from children of a previous marriage. This is to ensure care when there is the need for such. And adoption is important in Middle Babylon where a text records the adoption of a girl by a woman, presumed to be an elderly widow, and who is preparing for the time when she may need care. In the meantime, the adopted daughter, says the author, will either be given in marriage or work as a prostitute. Note that the elderly woman seems to be acting legally independently. The 'daughter', if married, her husband will help maintain the widow, or her income as prostitute will do the same, says Rivkah Harris (1992). If the old woman makes her a slave, she is to return to her father's house, as free, because as a slave she is not entitled to inherit. This, however, does not mention the practicalities of 'taking care of' in the various ailments of old age such as care of the body, the grooming, toileting, dressing, feeding, for example. Was that left to slaves?

I'm tempted to emphasize the concept of 'fictive kin' here. This is a useful catch-all concept for adopted kin, or close neighbours, or maybe also care workers. None of these 'belong' to the elderly in terms of blood relationship so why should they be described in kinship terms? Perhaps the focus is on major and much-needed assistance, and perhaps on type of relationship. The assistance we can guess, but just what kind of relationship might the fictive kin have. Warm, affectionate, responsive? Appreciative? Intimate, in terms of physical and emotional care? If the latter, could we also then include slaves in the term 'fictive kin'? The informal care of many Egyptians fell to the part of servants, and sometimes slaves, at least for wealthier people. In a society with low life expectancy, slaves might become the only family someone had:

> I have taken them, I have fed them, I have brought them up. I have reached this day with them and they have done me no harm. They have rather treated me well. I have no son, no daughter apart from them. And if I have fields in this country, if I have goods in this world,.... these shall divided between my four children, Padim being one of them. (from an Adoption papyrus Year 27 of Ramses XI)

Care-Hands-on

So what did hands-on caring consist of? and when the cared-for older person died, what happened to their carer?

Physical caring at a guess would be by female adult children or if there were no children or none willing or able to care, then other women, such as a servant or slave-girl, might have been adopted on condition of caregiving until death of her owners/master and wife. These carers might have wondered what would happen to them after the death of the older person. The slaves were under conditions of 'paramone' a clause in a manumission contract, whereby a slave had to do the work required, but was semi-free, in that he/she would be completely free after the work was completed. For example, two 'daughters' so-called (but one might have been a slave-girl) were required to look after their 'mother' until her death. To ensure their freedom after her death she 'cleansed' them before the god Samas. Samas (or Shamash) was also known as Utu, and was the sun-god who was the enforcer of divine justice, and also took considerable interest in human affairs, aiding those in distress.'Cleansing' here presumably means freedom.

As a matter of interest here, when a slave-girl was 'freed before Samas' she was not allowed any inheritance after the death of the old woman for whom she cared.

Bodies were exceptionally important to the ancient Egyptians, with daily washing, scenting, and anointing as well as clean linen. Another important improvement for the elderly were remedies against grey hair, and cures against baldness. But, as Casson (1978) says, only the wealthier members of the population could do this, while peasants shaved their hair off, and the middle-classes did their own hair.

And teeth were cleaned and mouths freshened regularly. So presumably this was carried out for the disabled and sick elderly as well, remembering of course, the earlier comments on dentition and that there might have to be considerable mouth care, and care in feeding foods easy to masticate.

Another intriguing part of bodily care is the use of prostheses both for the living and the afterlife. Prostheses were generally of a cosmetic character, such as an artificial toe made of cartonnage at the British Museum or, as a preparation for afterlife, an addition such as a forearm on a mummy housed now in Arlington Museum in Barnstaple, England, and an artificial penis and feet on another mummy in the Manchester Museum. A wooden big toe prosthesis has also been found which must have improved the walking capabilities of its wearer, a fifty to sixty year old woman, who wore it after her big toe had been amputated, possibly because of gangrene. And there was a glass eye with a white eyeball and a black pupil, but lacking an iris, which was probably inserted into the empty eye socket of a mummy rather than used by a living person. The ancient Egyptians' belief systems obviously took care of the body in its journey to the afterlife, and living therewith, of course, the shabti to perform the tasks required.

There are other pragmatic forms of care in terms of orthotics—walking sticks, staves, limbs, and amulets are also mentioned, with magic potions to discourage the illness and hopefully restore and maintain good health. A form of spiritual caring, perhaps? These amulets were either made in the form of body parts, whose completeness could be transferred to the owner's body or as containers to hold inscribed spells to cure afflictions such as blindness. There were two paraplegic individuals, whose burials were excavated, who could only have survived wounds such as fractures and healed through nursing care.

However, these latter tend to be more formalized care, while the paraplegics may well have received family help and servant or slave help.

Abuse?

Was there abuse? Squabbling in the households? There might well be a degree of intergenerational tension, due to patterns of residence and inheritance. From experience and from some knowledge of other societies, I'd add caregiving to that. And this is supported by a discussion of abuse at Deir el-Medina. The legal sources are very clear. Two wills demonstrate that when family members were negligent, they could be publicly shamed and fiscally punished. Naunakhte was one public shamer as we have seen. When she drew up her last will, she said that she had brought up her nine children, given them everything appropriate to their position, but now that they were all grown, they did nothing to care for her. She disinherited one son and three daughters. One daughter remained to inherit, and of her Naunakhte said, 'She shall have her share in the division of all my property, except for the emmer-wheat, which my three male children and one daughter have given to me.' (Marie Parsons, https://www.touregypt.net/featurestories/oldage.htm).

In a second will, there was a 'reattribution of possessions' where Jmn-pA-hApi removes his wife from his will after she neglected him. A third, Pn-nbw neglecting his father/grandfather, was reprimanded by community officials in writing and was potentially excluded from burial rites, an act which would have forfeited his rights to inheritance.

And another story of abuse we can see in the Select Papyri, 2.268:

> To King Ptolemy greeting from Ctesicles. I am being wronged by Dionysius and my daughter Nike. For though I had nurtured her…when I was stricken with bodily infirmity and my eyesight became enfeebled she would not furnish me with the necessaries of life. And when I wished to obtain justice from her in Alexandria…she gave me a written oath by the king that she would pay me twenty drachmae every month…Now, however, corrupted by that bugger Dionysius, she is not keeping any of her engagements to me, in contempt of my old age and my present infirmity.

It seems we have here a clear case of elder abuse here, documented by Peregrine Horden and Smith (1998).

So, elderly abuse certainly existed and documentation shows the very public punishments for such abuse. Presumably, such public shaming of this communal response to neglect would force/motivate family members to take care of each other.

Care-medical

No doubt individuals will choose their own way of doing things, including care, but there are still certain systems which inhabit the caregiver's environment. Abuse introduces us to one of the formal systems of care, that of legislation, and its recognition of the role of caregiver with its duties and appropriate actions.

And to continue our discussion on formal systems, if we go to 3000 BC we will find the beginning of the medical records in the Egyptian healthcare system. Egyptian society was the first to classify medications and also to develop plans to maintain people's health. These health and care systems also involve hygiene: a ritual hygiene through washing with pure water in a temple ensures both physical and religious protection against disease. And medical texts of the time describe methods to purify a space, and also objects in daily life, to seal and protect from contaminants. Such treatment would decontaminate and purify beds, which could indeed house contaminants.

Herodotus in fifth-century BC has described the highly specialist system of medicine in an ancient Egypt with each doctor being responsible for the treatment of only one disease: 'So each doctor treats only one disease and the whole place is crammed full with doctors. Some are oculists, others deal with head complaints, others are dentists, others deal with stomach trouble.' Apparently Egyptians took care of themselves with purgatives and emetics and cleared themselves out for three days running once every month.

Egyptian doctors were considered to be the best in the ancient world of the time, says Herodotus, and certainly on reading the sources, there are not only lists of problem issues but also lists of the professionals dealing with these.

The question here is: did the doctors instruct the caregivers, how did caregivers receive their instructions and what was the interaction between the two? I recommend a return to the African article of Elhabashy and

Abdelgawad. Doctors used males as helpers. Females were confined to midwifery, baby care, and wet-nursing.

So gender becomes an interesting element here. Men were the nurses, it seems.

Another interesting element in the medical scenarios could be that of slavery: an exchange of labour for protection (Pargas and Schiel 2023). Could part of this labour be that of caregiving within the medical scene as well as giving care in people's homes?

Care-spirituality, Ma'at [Balance]

We have looked at the demonology behind diseases, now we come to the powerful gods and goddesses who focus on correct behaviour and morality.

So behind the health and medical experts were, of course, the gods and goddesses. There is considerable complexity in the Egyptian system of gods and goddesses, who were seen not only as the lords of creation, but also as the custodians of order, and also to be considered as friends willing to help and guide the people of the land. In particular, there was Heka, who, among other duties, was the power which enabled the gods to perform their functions and allowed human beings to commune with their gods. He was all-pervasive and all-encompassing, imbuing the daily lives of the Egyptians with magic and meaning, and sustaining the principle of *ma'at* upon which life depended.

This principle of *ma'at* [balance] infused the care system with a sense of correct behaviour and morality. For our particular focus, we have to note that should there be transgressions against these forces of order, then all sorts of dire things would happen, including children abandoning their elderly parents and even after death, the influence would continue, as shown in a papyrus letter dated around 1250 BCE (AI mode).

'One example of influence from the dead is a complaint from a widower's writings, who wrote to his dead wife saying he had taken good care of her, and he blamed her for his current misfortunes, but he had had a good doctor to attend her and had given her a good funeral. He had not married again. Therefore he expected that her influence would be more beneficial than it obviously was. His good care was expected to achieve results as in positive relationships, even after death. Generally, people were expected to act with honour and truth in matters that involve family, the community, the nation, the environment, and the gods. And that surely included giving care.

From Mesopotamia are a number of stories showing care systems, and we are still into the spiritual. The Babylon creation myth, Enuma Elish shows a changing relationship between young and old, where older gods object to the aggressive, boisterous behaviour of the younger gods. The relationship with the aggressive behaviour of the young creates a source of conflict: the old want to rest by day and sleep by night; the young want to dance and play. But, then, along comes the young god Marduk. He creates a stable order and structure of the universe, including sanctuaries and offerings. The result is that the old then turn (I'm not quite sure how), from being productive towards receptive.

It's a good story! Yet again, there seems to be a morality, likely to be universal, whereby the emphasis is on the young caring for the old, through the medium of religious sanctuaries and offerings.

Caregiving makes its appearance here, and maybe we can link it in with the notion of balance. Could we argue that care provides a balance for the older person, to link the older person with the norms of society in terms of hygiene, care of the body, feeding, maybe socializing. It's hard to know exactly what form care might take for each individual, but perhaps dealing with the practicalities of various care needs will restore that balance. In fact, I suggest that restoring and maintaining this sense of balance is one of overall significance within the carer role. To create, maintain, and sustain a sense of harmony and connectedness to people and places, to the spiritual and the practicalities of daily living, is something which might be kept in mind in caregiving in general. The spirituality of balance, is discussed in Egypt in particular, with the god Heka, the goddess Ma'at and the health god Sekhmet predominant.

It seems that everyone was responsible for maintaining the balance in the universal order. If only one transgressed, then there was chaos, and chaos opposed everything the Egyptians knew and valued. If chaos reigned, then the realm would be in terror, and in Egypt, the sun would not rise, the Nile would not flood, crops would not grow, and children would abandon their elderly parents.

Conclusions

Looking back at the health systems of ancient Egypt, consider what the elderly must have faced. Egyptians had complex and even ambivalent attitudes towards deformity, but it seems that mostly they treated the sick and disabled with kindness and humanity. The *Instruction of Amenemope*, one of the Wisdom texts giving a moral and ethical code on how to behave, tells society how to treat the lame, sick, or insane and that since these were the creation of the gods, they should be respected. However, if there was such instruction, then it was clearly required, because treatment of the disabled (and this could include the elderly) was not ideal. As well as the spiritual, we have the legal system insisting on reciprocity the legalized transference of property and wealth is clearly written in the wills of wealthy people. Direct inheritance is important, but also so is the ability to disinherit, should care not be forthcoming. And in the case of the adoptees, the inheritance is also a legal document. The pragmatics of need and care are emphasized in these legal documents. So when we think in terms of reciprocity, then as far as inheritance is concerned, children-daughters as well as sons-inherited all possessions from their parents. For example, one man named Nekhtefmut, a priest of Amun during the 22nd Dynasty, handed over his properties to his daughter during his lifetime, in recognition of the fact that she had taken care of her parents in their old age (https://www.touregypt.net/featurestories/oldage.htm).

In fact, property and wealth, for the well-off Egyptians, are basic components in care-receiving and caregiving: reciprocity in what can be given on each side is important and part of making sure of care is to provide the inheritances as needed, required, or to hold them in abeyance to ensure good care.

As well as healthcare systems and the spiritual underpinnings of society where we have seen some confrontation by demons, there is a debate on whether the public system of palace or temple of the time acted also as a welfare system substitute for family care. It ensured that there were rations, though reduced, for men without children, and these were at the same level as for weaned children who were too young to work. What about the elderly in need? Were they also cared for in this way?

Another interpretation of reduced rations given to old and handicapped members of work teams by neo-Babylonian temples is that this indicates a sign of reduced production and those people no longer able to work dropped out of the list altogether, the burden of care being shifted to their families. However those without families, that is, without children, do seem to have been given some rations.

This is a question that requires further study in the extensive institutional archives of both periods. However, if we consider the practice of neo-Babylonian temples in acquiring aged servants, at the end of their master's life, as permanent temple slaves, it seems possible that the temples might have a social welfare role even though there are some queries about the temples' social welfare role as the ultimate refuge of the destitute elderly.

In conclusion, provisions for the elderly varied greatly from class to class and even from family to family. The wealthy had their ways of drawing an income from their estates, requiring little effort or supervision on their part; they might also be granted an official called 'staff of old age' to fulfil the more onerous duties of office, while the senior partner retained the title and presumably much of the salary Those who were less well off depended on their children for support, and there is good evidence of working arrangements between parents and offspring.

Some writers, like those for the Neanderthal, have indicated how risky they believe it to generalize from ancient texts, and these writers have pointed this out, as we have already discussed. After all, it may be that individuals arrive at their own, sometimes highly personal, solutions to problems like how to take care of an aged parent.

To complete this chapter I want to take from Stol and Vleeming (1998) a unique text on caregiving (perhaps indicating a reciprocity) the Amara stela, in which a woman is given the entire inheritance of her brother and mother with which to maintain herself and their mother.

> Statement of the Second Prophet Hori: he says "As for all the property of the Overseer of the Granary Paser, our father, consisting of fields in the country, slaves, female, and trees (?) they belong to the Songstress of Khnum Irytekh from son to son, heir to heir". Statement of the Songstress of Horus, Lord of Aniba, Tamehyt: she says "As for all the accumulated wealth that the Overseer of the Granary Paser made for me, it shall be given to Irytekh, my daughter; it is she who will make an old age for me." (p. 220)

Is this because the son did not want mother, did not need the inheritance. And in the phrase 'making an old age' is this a unique reference to the physical care for an ageing parent?

The questions increase. Horden and Smith (1998) challenge a golden age of caregiving. And they are right. But we have ideas to add to our carerscape: formal and informal systems of care such as spirituality, with some emphasis on facing illness demons, family, slaves, household and 'fictive kin'; legality from contractual details on care; spatiality, houses, rooms, beds, bedding, noise, odours. And perhaps we can add 'balance' within the care situation, to maintain connectedness to daily life.

The last words in this chapter remain with Stol and Vleeming (ibid.) concluding that provisions for the elderly varied greatly from class to class and even from family to family.

And the total amount of documentation on the subject of care for the elderly remains small, however, reflecting its family context. Perhaps too, this is yet another subject so familiar to the Egyptians themselves that did not need to write about it. We often know the least about the most common features of daily life (p. 221).

The journey continues.

References

Aboth or 'The Fathers,' otherwise Pirk'e aboth, "Chapters of the Fathers': a treatise in the Mishnah consisting of maxims and aphorisms of ancient 'fathers' or rabbis: analogous to the Book of Proverbs in the Old Testament. africame.factsanddetails.com/article/entry-202.html-section

Allam, A.H., M.A. Mandour Ali, L.S. Wann, et al. 2014. Atherosclerosis in Ancient and Modern Egyptians: The Horus Study. *Global Heart* 9 (2): 197–202. https://blogs.ucl.ac.uk/researchers-in-museums/2015/03/02/old-age-in-ancient-egypt/.

Brewer, Douglas J., and Emily Teeter. 2007. *Egypt and the Egyptians*, 2nd ed. Cambridge: Cambridge University Press. https://fathom.lib.uchicago.edu/2/21701778/.

Casson, Lionel (1978) Ancient Egypt: Great Ages of Man, Time-Life Books.

David, A. Rosalie, Amie Kershaw, and Anthony Heagerty. 2010. Atherosclerosis and Diet in Ancient Egypt. *The Lancet* 375 (9716): 718–719.

Elhabashy, Samad, and Elshaima Abdelgawad. 2019. The History of the Nursing Profession in Ancient Egyptian Society. *The International Journal of African Nursing Sciences* 11: 100174.

Forshaw, R. J. 2009. Dental Health and Disease in Ancient Egypt. *British Dental Journal* 206 (8): 421–424. https://www.nature.com/articles/sj.bdj.2009.309

Harris, Rivkah. 2003. *Gender and Aging in Mesopotamia: The Gilgamesh Epic and Other Ancient Literature*. Norman: University of Oklahoma Press.

Horden, Peregrine, and Richard Smith. 1998. *Locus of Care, Families, Communities, Institutions, and the Provision of Welfare Since Antiquity*, 1st ed. Comparisons and Continuities from Antiquity to the Present, 21. Oxfordshire: Routledge, 2014.

Laisney, Vincent Pierre-Michael, 2007. *L'Enseignement d'Amenemope*. Studia Pohl 16 (Pontifical Biblical Institute).

Janssen, Rosalind, and Jac J. Janssen. 1996. *Getting Old in Ancient Egypt*. London: The Rubicon Press.

Leek, F. 1996. *"The Dental History of Manchester MUMMIEs", quoted in Ana Maria Rosso* Dentistry in Ancient Egypt, Qeios.

Lucarelli, Rita. 2011–12. Demonology During the Late Pharaonic and Greco-Roman Periods in Egypt. *Journal of Ancient Near Eastern Religions (JANER)* 11: 109–125.

Lucarelli, Rita. 2013. Ancient Egyptian Demonology, Radical Matters Editions Label, www.radicalmatters.com. Èskathon.

McDowell, Andrea. 1998. Legal Aspects of Care of the Elderly in Egypt to the end of the New Kingdom. In *The Care of the Elderly in the Ancient Near East Brill*, ed. Marten Stol and Sven Peter Vleeming, 210–213. Brill: Leiden.

Palgrave Handbook of global slavery throughout history (2023) Dokumen Pub.

Pahhotep (2388 BC). The Teachings of Ptahhotep—http://www.peuplesawa.com/

ParsonsMarie. https://www.touregypt.net/featurestories/oldage.htm

Parsons, Marie, Old Age in Ancient Egypt in Tour Egypt, https://www.touregypt.net/featurestories/oldage.htm.

Apocalyptic Aperiodic serie | Philosophical working Papers | An E.book based anthology of philosophical essays, articles and essays in literary, non-literary and extra literary types, regarding apocalyptical, hermeneutic, escathologic and hermetic topics.

Roth, Martha T. 1987. Age at Marriage and the Household: A study of Neo-Babylonian and Neo-Assyrian Forms. *Comparative Studies in Society and History* 29 (4): 715–747.

Stol, Marten, and Sven P. Vleeming, eds. 1998. *Care of the Elderly in the Ancient Near East*. Brill: Leiden.

The-Instruction-of-Amenemope https://www.britannica.com/topichttps://www.attalus.org/docs/select2/p268.html. Select Papyri, 2.268

www.perankhgroup.com/indexhtm

http://cojs.org/mishnah_avot_5-21-_stages_of_life/

Other Good Reading

Foner, Nancy, quoted by Rivkah Harris in The Conflict of Generations in ancient Mesopotamian Myths (1992, October). *Comparative Studies in Society and History* 34 (4): 621–635.

Harris, Rivkah. 1992. The Conflict of Generations in Ancient Mesopotamian Myths. *Comparative Studies in Society and History* 34 (4): 621–635.

Pargas, Damian A., and Juliane Schiel, eds. 2023. *Palgrave Handbook of Global History: Slavery*. Cham: Palgrave Macmillan.

http://quatr.us/egypt/people/family.htm

Winkler, Elke-Meinrad, and Harald Wilfing. 1991. Tell el-Dab'a 6, Anthropologische Untersuchungen an den Skelettresten der Kampagnen 1966–69, 1975–80, 1985. Vienna.

CHAPTER 5

Soundings from Ancient Greece and Rome

Introduction

Since the two ancient societies of Greece and Rome are geographically close, often spoken of together and compared or linked in some way, it might be simpler to consider them together, looking at their similarities and differences. And soundings from them may give us further ideas for the carerscape. Some of the insights will be from their social systems, probably fewer will be from personal experiences, since due to the source material here we are still focused on more general systems of care than of the interpersonal relational aspects of care. But my interest in the latter remains, and where possible I want to highlight the personal individual care for those at home, describing caring individuals and groups, as well as the systems which mark out a caring society, if we consider the legalities and spirituality in these terms.

The timeline of these great societies is somewhat blurred, with Greece originating around 8000 BCE and ending with the death of Cleopatra in 31 BCE, with a Roman invasion in 146 BCE, marked as Greco-Roman period to the 30 BCE time.

So we have a big world with these two countries, an extensive period of time and a mixture of information, with diverse evidence of the experiences of ageing and everyday life, and inferred where possible through the bricolage of data about housing, hygiene, food, and general social interaction. Much of the evidence is textual, some information emerges from

B. Hale, *Historical Reflections on Care in the Western World*,
https://doi.org/10.1007/978-3-031-87128-3_5

different categories of artefacts, some from human remains and some is visual and observational.

Context

To place the elderly in context, let's try a little bit of historical visualisation. Let's imagine ourselves back into those ancient times, with narrow noisy streets, likely to be smelly to our nostrils, crowded houses for the poorer population, and with public latrines and baths. And we can move around observing how older people were treated, perhaps even detecting care being given if we can follow the disabled elderly to their homes.

Streets of both countries were crowded, houses of the wealthy were spacious with several rooms for specific purposes: store room, workroom, and bedrooms. In Greece there was a men's room for entertainment of male associates, and sometimes a separate entrance so that visiting men would not see/meet the women. Sometimes women had a special room, called a 'gynaikon'.

Housing for the poor consisted of small dark apartments; in Greece the apartments consisted of one, two, or at most, three rooms. In Rome, housing was close together in an insula, or a building which could house between 30 and 50 people, providing some neighbourliness, perhaps, and help if needed. For the wealthier Romans, the 'domus' was a single-storey house, with a courtyard and many rooms, including one for slaves. Depending on issues such as, for example, mobility, general infirmity, and perhaps need for bed rest, care in wealthier houses would most likely take place in the back rooms, the place of women and the slaves and servants. In the poorer apartments, of one or two rooms, care would take place wherever possible.

Furnishings meant stools and chairs, bed of a baseboard on four legs, or a stringed wooden frame, with pillows and cushions of wool, feathers, leaves or hay—or whatever material could be found. In the poorer houses, beds might be lifted in daytime, and replaced at night. In the wealthy houses were latrines, while poorer houses made do with pots to be emptied as needed.

Women's roles differed from place to place, and this is important to consider especially in terms of caregiving. For Greece, we need to look on Sparta and Athens as different entities. In Athens, the position of women was more restricted than that of the other areas. Many men refused to allow their wives to leave home; her job was to manage the household and the household slaves. Women lived in a separate part of the house, and even ate separately from the men. Their workforce consisted of slaves and servants whom they organized to help run the household and, let's assume this, to help care for the elderly. Of interest is that the poorer the woman, the more freedom she had to move out and about and, of course, to find employment, often as a servant or shop assistant. They were certainly unable to afford many slaves, so perhaps care of any elder relative would be for the more impoverished woman herself to undertake.

Life was different for the women of the city-state of Sparta. In Sparta, women were respected as the 'mothers of warriors'. Although they were not considered equal to men, they had more rights and freedom than the women of Athens. They were educated, played sports, could walk around the city freely, and were also able to own property.

Food looked magnificent, at least for the wealthier Greeks and Romans. Our information comes not only from recipes and menus, but from the visuals of vase paintings, wall frescoes, botanical and bone remains, archaeological artefacts and the architectural knowledge of pantries, kitchens, and dining rooms. Add to that the scientific detection of food residues preserved in dishes and storage vessels. From recipes, a selection of ingredients shows meat, eggs, fish, cheeses, olives, and many vegetables; likewise for ancient Rome there was a variety of foods, including: flamingo tongues, roast peacock and stewed snails and even dormice dipped in honey and rolled in poppy seeds.

But the poor of either culture failed to reach these culinary heights. In Greece they had locusts, black soup from pig's blood, coarse brown bread, dried vegetables and acorns, while in Rome the government provided free or cheap grain. This 'grain dole' was a bribe for popularity, apparently, and was used to make the porridge 'puls' the commonest meal for the impoverished. They would also be able to get bread and cheese but had very little meat.

This knowledge says little about what was fed to any invalid, or anything special for the elderly, but we can imagine sharing everything as much as was required and acceptable.

Hygiene and cleanliness were important. And these were as much social occasions as they were necessary for cleanliness. For the general public, the Greeks started to build bathhouses in their cities in the sixth century BC, constructing these next to the palaestra and the gymnasium. Vase paintings show various pools and also a form of shower and footbaths. Romans had good access to water, with magnificent public baths and commodious latrines, which allowed them to drop the waste into the water below, which was emptied eventually. Indoors, poor families used buckets or chamber pots, while wealthier families had their own latrines which drained into cesspits, with the waste eventually carried into rivers. Hygiene is always seen as a hallmark of Roman culture; but few, except wealthy, houses had any toilet systems, including drainage. Chamber pots used in the rooms were emptied out of a window when necessary and the resulting smells and diseases were undoubtedly unhealthy. Roman baths were for the more able-bodied who wanted to socialize. These baths had no individual drainage and had to be emptied. But Roman streets did have drainage systems and sewers, which carried away the detritus of the streets. Caregivers could be sure that whatever they threw out, would disappear.

Wiping the bottom after defecating varied—in Greece, shells or stones were used, in Rome various forms of 'wipes' were used until the advent of the communal sponge, which was cleaned after use by washing it in a bucket with water and salt or vinegar. Unfortunately this was insufficient to kill bacteria which then spread disease in the latrine. So although hygiene here was indeed attempted, it failed.

Along with the notions of hygiene we have the origins of modern medicine from two Greeks: Hippocrates and Galen, to be precise, and it's worth stating them here, so that we might have some inkling of treatment and perhaps even whether Hippocrates 'theory of the 'humors' influenced care. But that, I would have to say, is speculation. Hippocrates' theory basically states that the human body is made up of four substances, referred to as 'humors'. For ideal health, they had to be in perfect balance. To treat sickness, the humors had to be re-balanced. Galen's view was that an imbalance of each humor corresponded with a particular human temperament (blood—sanguine, black bile—melancholic, yellow bile—choleric, and phlegm—phlegmatic). And there is a description attached to each: individuals with sanguine temperaments are extroverted and social; choleric people have energy, passion, and charisma; melancholics are creative, kind, and considerate; and phlegmatic temperaments are characterized by dependability, kindness, and affection. Treatment, and presumably care, was intended to restore the balance of these humors.

And so we have the general context in which older people lived. For more information look up Robert Garland's works on disability and an interesting article by Philippe Charlier et al. (2012).

Elderly

How did these older people, especially those with disabilities and infirmities, live in these busy societies?

Particularly in Greece, it seems, there was a range of remarkably negative responses to infirmities and ageing, seen through the melancholic and derisory art and sculptures, the spiritual anger of the gods which caused the infirmities, and the pleading of Pericles to the Athenians to respect their elders. Many elderly shuffling around the streets were highly visible and became targets for unkind, jeering, and mocking behaviour. Roman humour as well as Athenian, laughed at physical deformity and ugliness. But perhaps many of the elderly kept out of sight since there was apparently considerable violence towards those with disabilities, and various authors write about how those elderly with disabilities were blamed and badly treated.

Surely these visible mobile elderly were the impoverished rather than the wealthier property owners. Writers of today, such as Tim Parkin (2003) describe older people in these societies more in terms of bodily and therefore highly visible changes. We are told of baldness, wrinkles, grey hair, loss of teeth, perhaps a faltering voice, forgetfulness, loss of certain mental characteristics, and possibly a shuffling gait too. Not that different from us these days, though premature hair loss in ancient Rome was culturally repulsive and to be disguised, to avoid mockery, while ageing baldness was also something to be mocked, and hair was in fact a prosthetic device, says Jane Draycott (2018) in writing about ancient prosthetics.

As well as street-visible targets convenient for derision, the weak and defenceless were portrayed in art as well. Rosemary Barrow (2018), cites an example of an old drunken woman avidly clutching a wine flask, such an image inviting derision as well as being lacking in compassion (pp. 62–75). Also visibly lacking in compassion are the sculptures of old men which demonstrate the pathos and infirmities of old age.

Why was there so little compassion? What lies behind this vehement dislike for imperfections? There was likely to be a supernatural cause, with disabilities and deformities seen in earliest times as an expression of the anger of the gods, and therefore requiring supernatural interventions. So says Temkin (1994) but, as he also says, such disabilities were increasingly seen as due to natural causes.

Such marginality produced anxieties and fear as Suzanne Dixon (1992) describes for Rome. She discusses the 'stereotypic laments' of the aged reflecting the near-universal anxiety that this stage of life would be characterized by neglect and want. And this brings us to care. Does care provide any support to improve this form of discrimination, or is it simply a case of maintaining the older person to continue living, even though on the edges of the society? In a poem about the hardship of a beggar's life, Martial (10.5.11 FF) depicts a derelict man in his dying moments. He hears dogs howling, anticipating eating his dead body, and he is trying, at the same time, to keep birds of prey (Noxias Aves) at a distance. He flaps his rags at the birds.

From Rome back to Athens and so far, the sources are general in their perceptions of visible ageing, disabilities and fears. However, there are contrasting perceptions and practices between Sparta and Athens. Athenians were required by law to look after their parents, but they were contemptuous of the elderly and this seems to have become a characteristic by the late fifth century BC. Sparta, on the other hand, held old people in high esteem.

In Xenophon's *Memorabilia*, Pericles despairingly demands, 'When will the Athenians respect their elders in the same way that the Spartans respect theirs instead of despising everyone older than themselves, beginning with their own fathers?'.

Herodotus in his Histories supports this description of the Spartans, claiming that deference towards older people is a characteristically Spartan virtue. If we want more vivid examples, he says that Egyptians and Greeks along with *neoteroi* will stand aside for the *presbuteroi* when they pass them in the street and rise when they enter the room. The Athenians apparently lacked such courtesies.

It is likely that respect engendered care, while despising and disliking would hinder care considerably. In fact, relationships might even be abusive and so different social recognition of the elderly might well influence how they are treated and cared for. As Karen Cokayne (2003) puts it:

> An old person could have status, authority and reverence, as long as societal expectations about how life should be lived were fulfilled. Respect for old age had to be earned. Whether or not an old man was able to fulfil his role in society depended largely on his social status, his own personal qualities and his physical and mental fitness. (p. 7)

So only the old, weak, decrepit, and those no longer socially useful, were marginalized by society. The question arises, of course, as to how these impoverished were cared for? Or were they cared for? We could infer that care of the marginalized and the mocked is more difficult than care for those who are respected and that perhaps there was a strong element of power.

Issues

Although the story is about the elderly, a good way to begin is by exploring problems of younger age groups, and *The Iliad* (Homer, c. 8th–seventh century BCE gives us vivid descriptions of many specific muscles, bones, and organs and the damage caused to these by battle wounds. For example, head wounds are described as lethal, while injuries to the limbs are not. For those interested, there are many articles detailing the wounds and their treatment described in *The Iliad*, including the management of these wounds and the treatment by therapeutic herbs. There seems to be little on the basic practice of caregiving, however.

As well as exemplifying medical practices and basic anatomical knowledge of the time, Homer also outlined the Greeks' spiritual outlook with regard to various ailments. At the beginning of the epic, the angered god Apollo strikes the Achaean army with a disease using his plague-spreading arrows. This sickness is characterized as highly contagious and quickly fatal, rapidly infecting the entire army. Only after the army offers a sacrifice to Apollo does he calm down and remove the affliction.

So placating the temper of the gods is one aspect of care or treatment, it seems.

It's more than probable that many Greeks and Romans, even before reaching old age, would have struggled with some disablement likely resulting from the demands and stresses of life in the ancient world. There are many descriptions of problems starting in middle age, such as failing eyesight and increasing deafness, also of rotting teeth. Back pains, ulcers, problems with bowel movements and bad feet. The range goes on.

What happened in middle age likely continued into old age, and perhaps for some there were changes from independence to increasing dependence. That would bring with it not only hands-on caregiving but also a different awareness and use of the surrounding environment of space and time, and no doubt of individual emotions of the caregivers as well as dependants. Perhaps also, these dependants required other personnel to help and advise, such as the wise women or doctors. So the questions are: depending on the need, where did care take place? In the back rooms? Somewhere offering privacy? Or is this a modern notion? Who did the necessary bodily care, assisting in its hygiene, its dressing and undressing, grooming, and mobility, attending to needs and requests?

And accompanying the experiences of dependency due to the various physical problems were the emotions of grief, depression, and misery, along with irritation with the ageing physical condition. At the same time, many of the causes for such emotional stress comes from the suffering and degradation inflicted upon elderly in time of war; the physical effects, of course, but also the witnessing of family members' suffering. The older population/family members stand by, helpless. One example is that written about in *The Trojan Women* Hecuba has to witness sacrifice of her daughter and slaughter of grandson. Enough to bring on any bout of irascibility, grief and depression, frustration and helplessness, breaking irascibility into a number of component emotions.

Where did problems come from?

Spiritual or supernatural influences were considered likely by many, but Hippocrates thought otherwise. Much has been written about his beliefs, medicine as a scientific profession based on natural sciences, detecting and preventing diseases as well as treating them, says Peter Heins (2022).

Obviously the question arises as to how far the supernatural influences on health could be said to influence the care? And therefore would spiritual care be required to improve or support the individual?

There were clearly numerous health problems. As well as those already listed, there were: paralysis, viral disease, the plague of course, meningitis, measles, mumps, scarlet fever, smallpox with side effects of deafness and blindness, and both the latter are also a consequence of ageing. One descriptive entry in the Hippocratic collection of *Aphorisms* comments: 'Old men have little warmth and they need little food which produces warmth; too much only extinguishes the warmth they have. For this reason, fevers are not so acute in old people, for then the body is cold.' An interesting set of observations, and it would be good to know who made these observations and based on what evidence.

In addition to the above, there are also problems stemming from maltreatment, stress, exhaustion, accidents, war, failure in food distribution, and environmental pollution. These undoubtedly exacted a heavy toll upon those in every age group.

Furthermore, let's not forget the traumas of broken bones which could result in permanent disability, and it is easy to believe that disorders of the legs and feet were physically traumatic since it often signalled the end of someone's working life. There were of course disabled slaves, and further, disabled war veterans as mentioned above. Wounds, breakages, injuries to the brain, or to the cervical vertebrae causing paralysis would have been widespread. For mental illness, the better medical writers were in favour of a strictly physiological causation, for which a remarkable battery of cuppings, pummelling, massages, purgatives, and diets was prescribed by one doctor or another. In fact, there seems to be little reference to mental illness in old age, and then it is only of the most casual kind. There is a brief section in Hippocrates' *Aphorisms*, enumerating the diseases characteristic of each age group: the list for the old includes catarrhal coughs, arthritis, nephritis, apoplexy, insomnia, failing sight, deafness, and a few others, but not dementia, whether it existed or not: 'I know no way to penetrate the almost total silence.' says Sir Moses Finley (1984), one of the greatest experts on antiquity.

And Garland (1995) another expert, says that for Greece no professional care was available for the bedridden and it would have been the slaves who tended those in bed. At the same time, among the poor, those who were most at risk of becoming disabled as a result of both sickness and injury were slaves.

Most of the above were problems which could be cared for, including, quite often, those of the slaves if the household could afford, and were willing, to do so.

But there were some medical issues which marginalised their sufferers. Any disabilities causing ugliness or scapegoat status required some form of treatment, or sacrifice. Garland (1995) whom I shall refer to frequently, gives considerable detail of these marginalised individuals. Physical bodily perfection or at least normality is to be admired. When it is lacking, then the individual may be mistreated.

CARE-Who?

Like the ancient Egyptians, caregiving in ancient Greece and Rome includes a number of different aspects: gender, position in household vis-à-vis the cared-for, and being already occupied with other roles. Caregiving was most likely gendered work, and the main attention has been on women as healers, says theologian Elaine Wainwright (2006). However, healing in these terms is more likely to be of a shorter duration than caregiving, and may not involve a longer-term relationship. What about the notion of care itself, which may be part of, but in our terms, different from healing? What did that work consist of?

From the contextual knowledge we have, we can begin to highlight different aspects of care, such as the legal and the spiritual. We can add kinship to these and we can suggest a general acceptance of the role by slaves. And from these we can often manage to infer details of the emotional care: affection, duty, and perhaps lack of duty for some. There was considerable emotion from the elderly revealed through reading the Roman wills of the times, and suggesting a sense of direction and power over their care and support (Edward Champlin 1991).

So who accepted and became involved with caring, bearing in mind that care is a highly complex area for investigation? Note that we have overall oversight as well as hands-on body care and assistance; domiciliary care, spatial, financial, community, spiritual, legal. So again the question arises: who provides the care? Physical care, and support for grief, stress, and anxiety—and perhaps I can introduce social care here too—might be parcelled up among different groups of people such as slaves, servants, immediate family, wider kin, neighbours, community, and society at large. Caregivers ranged from kin, to adopted kin, to servants, to slaves. And caregiving was not an easy task: there are comments on the 'irascibility' of the elderly, their suffering and degradation, expressed through Greek plays and poetry. Hesiod's story of Pandora is a prime example where Pandora, given to Prometheus' brother, opens a jar in her care, which contained a number of unspecified evils, including sickness and death. These were then released into the world, to ensure Zeus' vengeance on Prometheus for stealing fire.

However, first of all, care by kin is legislated for, in the codes of the time, of Sparta and Athens, as Finley (1981) said: 'Sons were held responsible for the maintenance of their parents and grandparents, and that was the end of the matter' (p. 404).

So, overall care and oversight of care was by kin, however that is defined; immediate, distant or adopted. Herodotus said the Greeks in general, regarded care of the elderly, or *geroboskia*, as a sacred duty, with the responsibility for this to be undertaken by children. Legally, sons were supposed to support their parents in old age. Note the word 'support', which could refer to financial help and help with food and housing as well as actual physical bodily care. Care in legal terms is described as maintenance and support, financial, housing, and sustenance. And such care must be overseen or at least visible to onlookers so that any abusive situation can be checked. Often, though, knowledge of informal domestic care comes only from its breakdown.

In Aristophanes' play, in *The Wasps*, we have a story describing caring in some detail. A feisty, stroppy old man gives as good as he gets but in the end he is overcome and has to accept care for his various issues: obsessional thinking, paranoia, hoarding, drunkenness, and his insults to his son's friends. In the first Act, the slaves concerned with the old man's care outline the failure of various treatments, such as counselling, medical treatment, and even travel to provide fresh ideas. Various kinds of care are being offered. It ends with the son, being a man of means himself, keeping the old man safe.

Kin care, no doubt.

The involvement of kin may also include strong reciprocal connections. Roman wills show details of inheritance. Possessions, estates, and money must be handed down to kin, and linked with this inheritance, are the obligations of kinship to 'care for', support, help, maintain the elderly. No 'care' then 'no gain' is how we could read these wills.

So important is the need to organise an inheritance, that when there is no kin, then kinship must be created and that 'fictive kin' has to deliver the care required. The creation of kin is worth repeating, to emphasize the enormous importance of kin care. Kinship was so significant in terms of possessions and property and succession, that adoption was the only resource/recourse for childless couples. And clauses in the adoption documents carried with them a measure of duty and obligation. The adoptee would have to signify willingness, and would have to agree to clauses in the adoption documents to recognise their obligation to the adopting person, to make sure they would look after such a person.

This suggests that care might be delivered as a duty, as a legal necessity, but it never remotely suggests affection. It hints at the emotions of need to get help, and the pragmatics of legal obligations, but not the day-to-day care, nor how this was delivered.

These measures were of course only for those with possessions and money to leave behind, as well as being able to 'buy' care. And Garland comments (1995) that for those without help there could be a rapid deterioration and unpleasant death.

In later antiquity, much of the population would live alone, in the big cities of Rome, Antioch, and Alexandria, and would die in isolation after becoming bedridden.

However, value of kinship and its duty emphasizes the legal aspects of care and its particular significance: that of ensuring the wished-for continuity of inheritances of money and property. Then, the significance of the morality and spirituality is clearly a blueprint for what people should do. Morality is legalized, kinship is legalized, and care is to be undertaken, as a duty and as a legal obligation.

In a North Jersey.com article on the internet *Freedom and Culture in the New World,* we find that knowledge of Athenian law spreads far and wide. Christopher Belitto (2017) has quoted Moses Finley on the legal and moral duties of sons to ensure legal care and protection for their elderly. Failure meant punishment, such as being debarred from holding public office. And such care and protection extended beyond parents to grandparents and even great-grandparents should they be alive. However, bad parents, such as those who had sent their sons out as prostitute or failed to teach them basic skills, were not protected in such a way. But any failure on the part of sons, and their fulfilment of duties meant that they would lose their rights as a citizen. A fate worse than death for an Athenian.

Obviously, this legal safeguard was essential since abuse cases and cases of neglect happened in ancient Athens. Because of the general social issues there of disrespect for older people, the Athenians used the law to enforce care and protection of ageing parents.

Athens, however, restricted protection (of parents) only to those parents who had taught their son a trade. But from Delphi comes a fragmentary inscription that anyone found guilty of failing to feed his parents was to be bound over and conveyed to gaol.

Hesiod in his poem 'Works and Days' has noted that there was considerable insecurity on behalf of the older people regarding the level of support which children would give to parents. He stated that one of the characteristics of the 'present' Age of Iron in its most degenerate phase would be the fact that 'men will not pay their parents the due reward for their rearing (In Threpteria). However, could this be a direct consequence of parental impairment? No one knows. If the elderly were senile, or perhaps, in our terms, 'cognitively impaired', Athenian law would limit their rights of control over their estates. Heirs would have to prove that parents could no longer deal with their affairs. Plato's recommendation in the Laws by Plato (11.929de) describes the problems: 'if a man becomes insensate owing to illness, old age or peevish temper and wastes his property, his son shall be entitled to bring an action against him'.

If convicted of senility by the court, then a man would be debarred from handling his estate and would have to dwell in his own *oikos* or home and family as a *pais* for the rest of his life—i.e. as a minor.

Athenian law and its ambivalence in the safeguards it afforded to the elderly required yet another legal safeguard, which was that the Athenian law code, like its Roman counterpart, had a provision restraining heads of families from wasting their estates if it could be proved by their heirs that they had lapsed into senility, a condition referred to as paranoia as Garland explores in the Greek Way of Life (1990).

He continues by quoting the case of the sons of Sophocles who dragged their father into court to have him declared incapable of managing his business affairs. The old poet, by then in his nineties, replied to the charge by reading out to the jury the play that he was currently working on, the *Oedipus at Colonus* and then disingenuously innocently inquiring, 'Does that play seem to be the work of an idiot?' The Athenians dismissed the charge!

In ancient Athenian society, elderly parents were extremely dependent on their offspring. Though fathers could charge their sons with criminal neglect, the latter in turn could accuse their fathers of senility. Moreover, since fathers were legally bound to leave their entire estate to their sons, they were not in a position to exert moral blackmail by threatening to disinherit them.

Fictive Kin

At the same time, many older people cared for by adopted kin enjoyed a longer old age, with the 'satisfaction of growing very old, good health and happiness' as a gift from the gods (Rivkah Harris, 2003).

Filial piety is clearly to be expected from fictive kin as well, and the evidence suggests that many such sons and daughters were devoted to their elderly parents. However such practice was not invariable, and ill treatment of parents came under the heading of impiety, a crime which the gods themselves would punish, as Mikalson (1987) tells us, for Athenian society. Never mind whether the gods would punish such impiety, society itself objected to the ill treatment of elderly parents. There were objections to a candidate for the office of councillor partly on the grounds that he mistreated his mother both during her lifetime and even after her death, another detail from Garland (ibid. p.157). Lykourgos, a prominent politician after 338 BC maintained, 'It is the greatest impiety not to pass our lives benefiting those from whom we have received the beginnings of life and those from whom we have received many benefits.'

Now to Rome, where we see that legal documentation is objective without overt emotionalism. But emotions did exist and this can best be seen in some of the wills from ancient Rome, described by Champlin (1991) as very public documents, and quoting strong expressions of emotion:

> What naturally catches the eye are the explicit expressions of emotion: the dearest, most affectionate, most pious (or most ungrateful) of children, the rarest (or most obnoxious) of friends, the most (or least) deserving of slaves, the most beloved of fatherlands. (p. 203)

How much of this intense emotion was a true expression of family feeling will be unclear. For some families they would be real, for others the phrases represented expected platitudes.

Bodily Care

Another step in the caring story is to discuss the practicalities of care, such as who carried out the care of the body.

Care takes place of the body, for the body, and on the body in many instances and the provision of such care could well include healing with its curative matters, and nursing, which might be identified as more specialised and skilful knowledgeable care. All these appear to involve families and particularly women, in terms of oversight, supervision, and sometimes hands-on, skilled care and healing. The old body in these ancient societies was the focus of three sets of skills and activities, a triumvirate of healing, nursing, and caregiving. And we could consider that an extremely powerful group of three.

However, a major subdivision for care of the body seems to lie between 'care' and 'healing' which has a sense of 'curative' and medically 'making better'. Healing requires its own special knowledge and skills and has its own set of definitions, including curative and medicinal, while nursing and caregiving have a stronger sense of maintenance and improvement but not necessarily in the curative sense.

Nursing, which has a familial sense of 'sister' in Turkish and Greek, may have skills and knowledge which caregivers do not possess, and the provision of nursing care throughout the centuries in early societies was clearly the role of families and especially of women, according to Theofanides and Sapountia-Krepia (2015). It is not entirely clear whether the idea of nursing care professionalises and perhaps distances the caregiver to some extent. Or perhaps it simply describes what some women do, a distinction between hands-on care, and the knowledge of herbal and other remedies. The distinction between therapeutic and hands-on tending seems to be blurred, with the latter more or less ignored. But as Theofanidis and Sapountia -Krepia state in their historical overview, on the first page, 'Nursing has now become an independent scientific discipline with discrete evidence based knowledge but certainly the care side still has powerful historic, cultural and traditional roots'.

As well as healing, nursing, and caregiving, care also includes relational power. In fact, much of what I have gleaned focuses on gender rules, and maintenance of the power of men. Women caring for men suggests that these women are more powerful than the man, and this is unnatural. It was important that no woman be 'in charge' of a man as Helen King (1991) writes in a section entitled Power and Control (p. 19ff) in a chapter on nursing in the past:

> Care or nursing or any movement, which signifies the power of woman over man, is to be interpreted as unnatural. Although Demosthenes emphasizes the value of women's care you yourselves know how valuable a woman is in illness, being there to help a sick person.' Helen writes, in Pat Holden and Jenny Littlewood's work (1991) on nursing and anthropology, that any reference to women helping the sick is not straightforward. Women caring in sickness can take advantage of an unnatural position of control over a male. To be noted, too, is the comment that a woman can make poison as well as drugs.

An example of such power is demonstrated by Helen King (ibid.) in a description of the visit by an estranged wife and her mother to a quarrelsome husband. 'They came to his home bringing 'things suitable for the illness' and they 'watch over' him' (p. 13). There is no mention of any healers being summonsed, although the patient is so ill. In fact he is so ill that 'his sickness, his childlessness, the care [*therapeia*] of the women and his enmity towards his own kin' persuade him to recognise as legitimate his son by his estranged wife. This can also be interpreted as there being some manipulation involved.

But at the same time we should not forget the power the cared-for with his/her needs has and Garland in supporting the concept of family care brings in not only the strength of the carer position but also its burden. For the 'vast majority of the disabled' they were 'dependent on the goodwill and charity of their families', and no doubt were the 'victims of silent recriminations at the very least', considering that time taken out of earnings to give care would damage the personal and family economy.

The other major recourse for caring is slaves, many of whom could be bought in to care for the elderly. So says Christopher Xenopolous Janus writing in The Hellenic Communication Service (www.hellenic) that eclectic writer. Slaves giving care, and then women as overseers of care at least, were those most involved, and presumably more of the power lay with the overseer of care rather than the slave.

Other authors talk of the ordinary work of the house being done by slaves, and I am tempted to infer that this 'ordinary work' includes the mundanities of caregiving for the elderly. The cleansing and grooming of the body, the removal and disposal of waste products, perhaps feeding the disabled—could all be carried out by slave labour. The actual actions of care such as cleansing, removing waste matter, perhaps helping to walk, dress, bathe, and toilet, were performed most likely by slaves, according to Garland again. Domitius Tullus who, from all sources, sounds a most unpleasant individual, had to be turned, fed, cleansed, mouth cleaned—perhaps he had reason to be unpleasant? And this work was undertaken by slaves.

Spatiality

Bodily space has been dealt with in the details of everyday living but what could be introduced here is the use of prosthetics. Not only do these provide the body with the ability to move, hold, lift and move in some way, but also a prosthesis balances the body and provides it with a more normal stance and movements. Iron hands, legs, toes were those most often used for soldiers or former soldiers who lost a limb during wartime—but these soldiers can age, too, and the prosthesis is useful for their continuing independence. Definitely a task for the caregiver is assistance with prosthetics.

The other task for a caregiver is the use of 'conveniences' for incontinence. In the earlier days of these societies in antiquity, treatment of incontinence was by exercise regimes, in the baths and gymnasiums of both countries, according to Hippocrates and Galen. The Egyptians had devices for the collection of urine in males and pessaries for women so it is likely that these also were available in Greece and Rome. Incontinence therefore, for those who could afford such devices, was therefore manageable, and—as an important note—there was no need to change sheets or bedding of any sort, while with the poorer families, it is likely that the bedding would become soaked, and foul-smelling (at least to our nostrils) and though sweetened as far as possible with scented herbs, might have to be changed whenever the household could afford to do so.

So the household as a place of care is intriguing, considering the actual space of care as front or back of house, the type of bed and furnishings, and the necessaries for hygiene.

From such a brief discussion of housing and households we have some view of space and care, including the philosophical as well as the visual.

Space has many words added to it to specify what it is and also indicate what happens in that space. We can have living space, private space, public space, personal space, and shared space, all of these words indicating the use of that space. What needs to be highlighted also is caring space, the space where care, depending on what it is, takes place. This could be on the body as in the space of the body itself, as we have seen with prostheses and 'conveniences' or with the ageing infirm body in the space(s) which it can use, and how such space is used. This introduces the question of temporality as well, both for the cared-for and the caregiver: how much time is needed for different tasks, and how much time a caregiver has to focus on care only.

The question is also: what space did the families occupy and was there a specific use for different spaces, including that of caregiving, of course. Often in antiquity, the wealthier large families lived in the same house, from grandparents to siblings of parents, to children. There was a move from the multi-functional one- or two-room house to a multiple-room house, where functions can be distributed over different areas of the house, and individual rooms can have separate access. In fact, much can be inferred from the changes from a multi-functional room to a multiple-room house and a sick person could be confined to one room.

The possibility is that these changes are linked with the concept of privacy and perhaps a new and more private approach to life, since the residents within the house had more rooms, each of which could be reached separately. Generally, it seems to be that back spaces are women's spaces and domestic space. Front of house is communal, social, and men's space. So it is most likely that caregiving took place at the back, which suggests not only a certain sense of privacy but also a sense of invisibility.

Use of space is extremely important in caregiving, particularly that of beds and bedding, and the question arises: who slept where and how did they sleep? Singly or sharing bed space with a number of others?

Wainwright (ibid.) says rightly that this should form a specific study in its own right. In a fascinating comment she considers the concept of space as a force for healing in its own right.

Spirituality

Further aspects of caregiving which need to be considered include spirituality and the emotions in caregiving, and a consideration of the effects of power. These are undoubtedly influential in caregiving, perhaps on an individual basis rather than an overall direction, and will certainly add to our knowledge of the role and status of caregiver/nurse. As she says

> an ecology of healing emerges in which the other-than human, the air, water, space and diet, accompany the work of the divine healers towards transformation and healing. (p. 187)

Spirituality, which, like the legal codes, can provide a little information on different features of care, is in the realm of the different gods and their orders and demands, although the specific gods for the elderly are described in gloomy terms. Geras, the Greek god of old age, is depicted as a hobbled, thin, defenceless, vulnerable, and wrinkled fellow whom we would see as worthy of pity more than worship or fear. There are hardly any depictions of older goddesses at all. But one especially stands out by its negativity. In Hesiod's *Theogony*, we read about the birth of the gods. There, Night is named as the mother of Old Age, who is described as sad and accursed.

Nonetheless, the Greeks sought help from the divine. Until the sixth and fifth centuries BC, healing was rooted mostly in religion and magic.

Treatment and comfort was sought from priests, people offered sacrifices and prayers to certain gods and tried out medicinal herbs, and some tried out different traditional rituals. So care would involve the spirituality of the people being cared for. Tributes and votive offerings also went to Asclepius, and when the plague broke out in 430 BC, Telemachos of Archanes brought across a sacred serpent representing Asclepius to Piraeus, then to the Acropolis, and established a 'diminutive sanctuary'.

We can comfortably infer, then, that care has a spiritual element where belief in the gods as helpers and a sense of maybe 'mind over matter' are part of the caring context.

And spiritual healing eventually became located in a temple, although this did not occur until the cult of Asclepius created Temples of Healing, with the major site being at Epidaurus where patients could spend a night at the temple, when they would be visited by the god in a dream, and subsequently priests would interpret the dreams and prescribe treatment. Epidaurus also accepted sick patients to give them sanctuary, and eventually a large structure of 180 rooms was built to house the dying.

And there are other examples. But the question remains for me is whether spirituality affected the general daily care given, strengthening it and supporting it perhaps by temple visits of caregivers or priestly visits to the sick.

Power

And beyond the power of spirituality lies the power of the secular, already mentioned. It has to be asked: how was this power exercised and how was it monitored?

Presumably the benefactor warned/told the caregiver or would-be caregiver that he/she would inherit if care was forthcoming. Some individuals might continue to mention the inheritance factor when care was being given. But should caregiving not be as the cared-for wanted, how did he/she contact someone to remove the benefits from the will?

Elder abuse was obviously alive and well in ancient Greece. A revealing comment by Robert Garland demonstrates this: 'By the early fourth century contempt for the elderly had widely come to be perceived as a distinctive feature of the Athenian national character and one which sharply distinguished it from its Spartan counterpart…' (p. 99). Xenophon's *Memorabilia* (3.5.15) has Perikles demanding despairingly,

'When will the Athenians respect their presbuteroi the way the Spartans respect theirs, instead of despising everyone older than themselves, beginning with their own fathers?' Garland, again, says 'the most despised group were those in employment with other Greeks, whether on a permanent or on a temporary basis.' This may well apply to family carers, whether women in the family or slaves.

We can move to ancient Rome, if we wish, with remarkably similar results where Cicero demonstrates the ancient Romans' perceptions of ageing in *Cato Maior de Senectute*, where he concedes (3.8) that 'old age cannot be easy in extreme poverty' and he continues:

> And, indeed, when I reflect on this subject I find four reasons why old age appears to be unhappy: first, that it withdraws us from active pursuits; second, that it makes the body weaker; third, that it deprives us of almost all physical pleasures; and, fourth, that it is not far removed from death… To the old age of Appius Claudius was also added blindness. (para 16)

In conclusion, we have a rather mixed perspective on ageing and possibly also on caregiving in these ancient societies. Starting with the marginality of the elderly, ancient Greece and Rome demonstrate various systems of caregiving, from the systematic legalities and spirituality to the nuances of a frail elderly cared-for relationship where power and abuse can be perceived. At the same time, though, the insistence that there must be care and the means whereby those without kin can create a 'fictive' kin structure is a positive move in terms of care taking. And from the construction and use of prosthetics, and the existence of continence products, societies demonstrate an awareness of the body, its aesthetics and its balance. As usual, of course, is the distinction between the wealthy and the poor, and again as usual, care seems to be by women and likely by some slaves.

So to continue constructing the carerscape, there are the following ideas and vocabulary: kin, fictive kin, slaves, bodily care, spatialityand spirituality.

References

Barrow, Rosemary. 2018. *Gender, Identity and the Body in Greek and Roman Sculpture*. Cambridge: Cambridge University Press.

Bellito, Christopher M. 2017. *Honoring the Elderly: A Cautionary Tale from Ancient Greece*. North Jersey.com

Champlin, E. 1991. *Duty and Emotion in Roman Wills, 200BC–AD250*. University of California Press.

Charlier, Philippe, Luc Brun, Clarisse Pretre, Isabelle Huynh-Charlier. 2012. Toilet Hygiene in the Classical Era. *British Medical Journal* 345 (7888): 41.

Cokayne, K. 2003. *Experiencing Old Age in Ancient Rome Routledge Classical Texts*. Psychology Press.

Demosthenes Against Neaira Fifty-Ninth Speech, or An Appolodorus Speech.

Dixon, Suzanne. 1992. *The Roman Family*, 155,156. Baltimore and London: John Hopkins University Press.

Draycott, Jane. 2018. ed. *Prostheses in Antiquity*. Taylor and Francis.

Finlay, Moses I. 1981. *Economy and Society in Ancient Greece*, 157. London: Chatto and Windus.

Finley, Moses I. 1984. *Elderly in Classical Antiquity*. https://www.cambridge.org/core.

Garland, R. 1995. *The Eye of the Beholder, Cornell Univ* (p. 99). Press.

Harris, R. 2003. *Gender and Aging in Mesopotamia: The Gilgamesh Epic and other Ancient Literature*. University of Oklahoma Press.

Heins, Peter. 2022. Hippocratic Medicine's Principles form the Sophisticated Modern Medicine. *Perspective* 8 (2).

Herodotus, Herodotus. 1947. *The Histories. Translated by George Rawlinson*, 99. New York: Modern Library.

Hesiod Works and Days 187.9 cf. Thgn.821. (Pliny. Ep. 8.18) Hesiod Works and Days 187.9 cf. Thgn.821

Horden, Peregrine and Richard Smith, eds. 1998. *Introduction, Locus of Care: Families, Communities*. Institutions, and the Provision of Welfare, Routledge imprint, Taylor & Francis.

King, Helen. 1991. Using the Past; Nursing and the Medical Profession in Ancient Greece. In *Anthropology and Nursing*, ed. Pat Holden, Jenny Littlewood, Routledge, Library Editions.

Kolowski-Ostrow, AnnOlga, https://www.brandeis.edu/magazine/2013/spring/arts-and-culture/roman%20smells.html (3.5.15).

Leonard, John. 2017. *Sacred Hospitals of Ancient Greece*. https://www.greece-is.com/snakes-dogs-and-dreams/.

Martin, Thomas. 1996. *Greece: From Prehistoric to Hellenistic Times*, 2nd edn., 1996, p. 175. Yale University Press.

Mikalson, Jon D. 1987. *Athenian Popular Religion*. University of North Carolina Press.

Temkin, Owsei. 1994. *The Falling Sickness: a History of Epilepsy from the Greeks to the Beginning of Modern Neurology*. John Hopkins University Press, Baltimore and London.

Theofanidis, Dimitrios and Despina Sapountzi-Krepia. 2015. Nursing and Caring: an Historical Overview from Ancient Greek Tradition to Modern Times in International Journal of Caring Sciences, September-December 2015, Vol 8, Issue 3 p. 791.

\Xenophon's Memorabilia: Hippocratic Collection of Aphorisms 1.14 and in Threpteria: Studies on Ancient Macedonia (2012), M. Tiverios, P. Nigdele and P. Adams-Veleni (Eds), Aristotle University, Thessalonica.

Wainwright, Elaine. 2006. Women Healing/Healing Women, The Genderisation of Healing in early Christianity, (ch.5) Equinox, London.

More Good Reading

Ault, B.A., and Nevett, L.C. 2005. *Ancient Greek Houses: Chronological*. Social Diversity, University of Pennsylvania Press, Philadelphia.

Finch, Jacqueline. 2011. The Ancient Origins of Prosthetic Medicine vol377, iss. 9765, pp. 548–549, The Lancet, KNH Centre for Biomedical Egyptology, University of Manchester.

Janus, Christopher Xeneopoulos J, in Hellenic Communication Service: Care for the Elderly: From Cannibalism to the Greek way. http://wwwe.helleniccomserve.com/quotethegreeks.html.

Lang, Franziska. 2005. Structural Change in Archaic Greek Housing, ch.5 in Ault, Bradley A. & Lisa C Nevett. Ancient Greek Houses: Chronological, Regional, Social Diversity University of Pennsylvania Press, Philadelphia.

Nissin, Laura. 2016. *Academic Dissertation, Roman Sleep: Sleeping Areas and Sleeping Arrangements in the Roman House*. University of Helsinki.

Parkin, Tim G. 2003. *Old Age in the Roman World: A Cultural and Social History*. Baltimore: John Hopkins University Press.

Roisman, J.J. and Edwards, M. 2019. *Against Leocrates*. Oxford University Press.

Schultheiss, Dirk, Introduction, https://www.ics.org/Publications/ICI_3/v1.pdf/historique.pdf.

CHAPTER 6

Soundings for Care By the Early Judeo-Christians

Timeline: 30 CE (death of Christ) to 327 CE (death of Constantine).

Spirituality and community care form the basis for care in this chapter. And while there will still be some focus on kin and domestic care, I want to introduce group care and the outreach from a Christian spiritual basis. The core here is simple. It is that of shared values of Judeo-Christianity influencing people towards providing care for those in need, and while I still aim to highlight the elderly at home with their various problems, the emergence of plagues demands that we expand our view. So I'm moving our gaze from the intimate domestic sphere and the elderly to the wider community and of a variety of people of ages usually unknown.

Judeo-Christianity, with their related core values, inaugurated a wider brotherhood of man, with the message of 'do unto others' no matter whether they were of the same ethnicity or not. This message spread across numerous cultures as Christianity itself extended its influence far beyond its original country, influencing care activities over and above what we have seen so far. Christian groups were in Judaea of course, then the movement advanced in Greece and Rome and spread further along the Mediterranean in the second and third centuries. The progress then was to various settlements in and around the Mediterranean Basin, Southern Europe, North Africa, Anatolia, and in the east, Christian groups reached the Caspian Sea.

B. Hale, *Historical Reflections on Care in the Western World*, https://doi.org/10.1007/978-3-031-87128-3_6

Such groups tended to maintain a low profile, in terms of following the customs of the people of each country in respect to clothing, food, and the rest of their ordinary conduct, but, says the Epistle to Diagnetus, in Chapter 5, without going into detail they display to us their wonderful and confessedly striking method of life.

This mission of the early Church made the Christians more visible not only to care for those in Christian congregations but also offering outreach, beyond the non-Christians, and to other cultures, out into the wider community. Eusebius (314 AD) noted in his ***Ecclesiastical History*** that while the heathen fled the plague at Alexandria, "most of our brother-Christians showed unbounded love and loyalty" in caring for and frequently dying with the victims.

Such outreach was well organised through groups. Later in the chapter, the groups of almanah, spoudaioi, parabalani, and in the next chapter, the beguinage too will all appear and demonstrate both how and what they did and, importantly, why.

Certain individuals stand out in directing this outreach of care. Basil of Caesarea, pastor and theologian, called on the wealthier members of his congregation in mid-fourth century AD. He exhorted them to give and support and help the starving and oppressed, as he had done himself, building a hospital for the poor and a clinic for lepers. In his Sermon to the Rich circa 368, he says:

> What answer shall you make to the judge, you who dress walls, but will not clothe a man; who spruce up horses, and overlook an unfashionable brother; who leave grain to rot, but will not feed the starving; who bury your money and despise the oppressed?

In the earlier stages of Christianity it seems from Biblical readings that spirituality was the single most important influence in the changing perceptions of the body and of different abilities/disabilities. There are undoubtedly Gospel readings to show the influence: for example, Matthew 25:35–40:

> For I was hungry and you gave me food, I was thirsty and you gave me drink, I was a stranger and you welcomed me, I was naked and you clothed me, I was sick and you came to visit me, I was in prison and you came to me… Truly I say it to you, as you did it to one of the least of these my brethren, you did it to me.

This is indeed a change from the Roman lack of compassion. According to the *Christian History Magazine* #101, compassion was not a well-developed virtue among the pagan Romans; mercy was discouraged, as it only helped those too weak to contribute to society. In the cramped, unsanitary warrens of the typical Roman city, under the miserable cycle of plagues and famines, the sick found no public institutions dedicated to their care and little in the way of sympathy or help. Perhaps a family member would come to their aid, but sometimes even close relatives would leave their own to die.

But for the Christian, says Tertullian, who lived around 200 AD, 'It is our care of the helpless, our practice of loving kindness that brands us in the eyes of many of our opponents. "Only look," they say, "look how they love one another".' He writes a defense of Christianity in his *Apologeticum. Discussed by Warren Smith in an interesting article*

And more, from St John Chrysostom, when he was Bishop of Antioch (386–97) over these twelve years he emphasized charitable giving:

> Do you wish to honour the body of Christ? Do not ignore him when he is naked. Do not pay him homage in the temple clad in silk, only then to neglect him outside where he is cold and ill-clad. He who said: "This is my body" is the same who said: "You saw me hungry and you gave me no food", and "Whatever you did to the least of my brothers you did also to me"... What good is it if the Eucharistic table is overloaded with golden chalices when your brother is dying of hunger? Start by satisfying his hunger and then with what is left you may adorn the altar as well.

So the message of love and care was much wider than our initial focus, and will of course include the elderly.

Ageing

Psalm 90:12 informed the work of noted anthropologist Barbara Myerhoff (1980): 'Teach us to number our days, that we may present to you a heart of wisdom.'

This verse is one which could be said to inform the cultures of Judaism and Christianity as to respecting the ageing and elderly population. Other perceptions of ageing are clear in both Old and New Testament texts which insist on 'honouring' the father and mother, 'that thy days may be long upon the land'.

More texts insist on the wisdom of the elderly, meditation by the elderly on ageing, their behaviour towards their descendants which is to be kindly and reverent in their behaviour, and to teach and demonstrate how to behave: 'love husbands, children, sensible, pure, workers, kind (for women),' says Titus 2:2–3 and also specifically for men: 'temperate, dignified, sensible, sound in faith in love and perseverance.' 'Timothy (5:1–2) outlines the behaviour of younger people. Older men are not to be rebuked, but to be appealed to as a father, older women as mothers.

What is clear from the above is that, in general, when living with kin, the elderly were both to respect and love and be respected and loved, and indeed cared for, whether by family and beyond them, by servants or slaves, whichever was immediately available.

The biblical view of ageing and old people is in total contrast to the utilitarian view. The Bible views the presence of old people in a community as a sign of God's favour. This is what the Lord says: 'I will return to Zion and dwell in Jerusalem… once again men and women of ripe old age will sit in the streets of Jerusalem each with cane in hand because of his age' (Zech. 8:4) and conversely, the absence of old people is a sign of God's disfavour. The Lord, the God of Israel declares: 'The time is coming when I will cut short the strength of your father's house so that there will not be an old man in your family line.' (1 Sam. 2:31). The biblical view of ageing and old people is in total contrast to the utilitarian view. The Bible views the presence of old people in a community as a sign of God's favour.

And who cares? According to the Apostle Paul, 'Children …should learn to put their religion into practice by caring for their own family and so repay their parents and grandparents for this is pleasing to God' (1 Tim. 5: 3–8).

David Richmond in *A Biblical Perspective on Ageing and Old People*, (from The Selwyn Foundation) provides further biblical principles which address this situation. One is financial: 'If one of your countrymen becomes poor…help him so that he can continue to live among you…do not take interest from him…' (Lev. 25:25). In the book of Deuteronomy, there are even more specific God-given instructions to the Israelite nation regarding the care of the destitute and elderly. For example in Deut. 24:19–22 we read that 'He commanded them to leave some of the grain, olive and grape harvest for 'the alien, the fatherless and the widow' (Also see Lev. 19:9–10, 23:22, etc.) The early Church took the sharing of resources very seriously. We read in Acts 2:42–47 that: 'All the believers were together and had everything in common. Selling their possessions and goods they gave to anyone as he had need.'

But was this always possible? When there were major problems, as in the impoverished groups, what happened? Were many older people living outside, perhaps pushed out of home because families were unable to cope? And we have the struggle with the plague for both elderly and younger. Information on the pagans tells us that Bishop Dionysius, living in Alexandria, describes how the pagans pushed the plague sufferers out, throwing them into the roads before they were dead. They treated unburied corpses as dirt, hoping to avoid spreading the disease, and to avoid contagion. But this was impossible, and the epidemics raged through the population, elderly and younger.

Issues

However, the familiar problems of ageing still existed, alongside the epidemics. With causal theories in mind, there is a list of the usual deformities ranging from a wide-angle view of the origin of disabilities and sickness to specific descriptions of disability and illness. Those include: blindness, deafness, arthritis, probably incontinence, and mental health disorders. And to these we can add the major epidemics of plague and leprosy. A considerable background of problems is outlined by Gary Ferngren (2009) who talks of shunning the chronically ill because of the demands made on the time and earning capacity perhaps of the caregivers. This chronically ill is certainly a wide age group of sufferers, but certainly the elderly will be represented. And Ferngren talks too of the abandonment of slaves 'on Tiber Island at Rome' where they might find some healing when they were old and useless. And then he comes to the elderly (people over 60) were who were sometimes left to fend for themselves, especially if they had outlived younger kin. Elderly were then often forced to live on the streets, in porches, on tombs or in makeshift dwellings.

Some of the bodily problems developed over a busy hardworking, and possibly undernourished lifetime. Some may well have been from birth. Like today there are the major illnesses, such as cancer and Parkinson's. In the past we have, as the sources describe, leprosy and the plague; there is some mention of measles—but, understandably, the sources dwell on the great epidemics of the times. More pragmatic information comes from Garland (1991, pp. 24–26/7) who discusses the basic types of illness/

disability experienced by many in the Greek-Roman world, and which no doubt continue into early Christian times. He quotes a Hippocratic treatise entitled *Aphorisms*:

> Difficulty in breathing, catarrh accompanied by coughing, problems of the urinary tract, arthritis, nephritis, dizzy spells, apoplexy, cachexia, itching of the whole body, insomnia, water discharge from the bowels, eyes and nostrils, dullness of vision, glaucoma and deafness. (3.31)

Further knowledge from previous societies suggest there is considerable osteoarthritis, with its advanced stage involving debilitating pain, gross deformity and, ultimately, virtual paralysis or more likely, possibly, immobility. Much of this information comes from works from authors such as Garland and Ferngren, discussing Roman Britain but there is some relevance to early Christianity, which I have included here because of its wealth of detail.

Further information from Ferngren (ibid.) also discusses problems among women, not always the elderly, suffering from iron deficiencies, because of poorer nutrition, which he says, occurred among about 41% of the women. Men were less affected because their diet was better than that of the women. The iron deficiency could also be attributed to malaria.

In addition, we have information, again from Garland (2010), that there were 'many malformations': club feet, Pott's disease, atrophy, and poliomyelitis.' (p. 45). We can see physicians attending to all the traditional illnesses: dermatosis, tuberculosis, nephritis, and hepatitis, along with a mention of blindness and certain epidemics. There are also talks of war wounded and victims of accidents.

To add to the above deformities, Garland talks too of a 'variety of viral diseases', e.g. meningitis, measles, mumps, scarlet fever and smallpox, and there is also some talk of debilities of slaves: injuries, crippled, 'bow-backed'. Such health issues can be attributed to maltreatment, stress, exhaustion, accidents, war, failure in food distribution and environmental pollution.

How did the society at the time perceive these issues? Either from spiritual/demonic influence or, from Hippocratic times, as environmental influences. The spiritual appears here again: although disabilities were not considered as coming from the gods or in this case God, nonetheless there was a sense of spirituality which influenced the disability. Amanda Porterfield (2005) writes that first-century interpretations of Jerusalem and

Jesus also drew on an older theme in Hebrew scripture that interpreted disease and misfortune as God's punishments for sin and disobedience of his law, and health and prosperity as blessings from God in response to repentance from sin.

However, it seems that the early Christians considered health issues to be the result of natural causes rather than demonic possession or divine punishment. Whether this makes a difference to the type and method of care is not clear.

What the sources give us is a list of disabilities and diseases. They also give perceptive words such as 'weak' and 'the poor', and 'deformities' and 'abandonment', and spiritual words such as 'demonic' and 'satanic'. These give some clue on general perceptions of illness and disability, but whether or how much these influenced care or not does not appear in the sources I have discovered.

And there was a move to care for the poor, a term which became descriptive of 'weak' and later, 'lower classes' who were seen as deserving the help which had belonged to 'the demos' or common people. This 'little noticed movement' in fact marked a huge change, 'one of the truly revolutionary changes in human sentiment in Western history' says Ferngren (ibid.). This insight surely indicates the changing times from classical to Christianity.

Care

And so we come to care itself— what, where, and how; why and who?

Sources are varied, of course. Frescoes, tombstone inscriptions, as well as documentation, all give some information.

The 'why', demanding respect for the elderly, we can see through the various religious injunctions in both the Old and New Testaments. Given these injunctions to respect older people, what did that mean in terms of practical care? The 'who' we can infer from looking at inscriptions on many tombstones, not necessarily accurate of course.

Who?

While the new element here is care by specially set up groups this is not to ignore the significance of family and household in supporting and caring.

Briefly, families, with their expansive membership and often involving a general household, are undoubtedly the first port of call for caregiving for their older people, as many writers have noted. David Balch and

Carolyn Osiek (2003) offer a multi-disciplinary view of these early families. including slave families and slaves in families, from Dale B. Martin (p. 207 ff). And of course the upper and wealthier classes have greater space to accommodate more members, including slaves and boarders.

Before we continue, though, perhaps we should define 'family' here. It might consist only of nuclear family, of course, but also can contain extended family members, including grandparents, and slaves. It could also contain adult children and their spouses. The family formed the 'basic constituent unit of ancient society'. It could also include non-biological kin as well as slaves, apprentices, and boarders, reinforcing the concept we have already identified, that of 'fictive kin'. But household rather than family is the word most often used and to paraphrase various historians,[1] the household or family are the 'chief locus of health care' as Horden and Smith have identified (2006).

Household could be coterminous with family, and also expansive in that it could include fictive kin, as in those adopted non-kin, slaves, apprentices, and boarders, all living within the same building. The definitions of 'household' can range between small and large units, with possibly several families living together, including grandparents, families of grown children, adoptees, perhaps divorcees, as well as slaves and other dependants. In some cases it might also include a labour force, and domestic animals. A different concept from 'family' clearly, but at the same time perhaps slightly closer to 'family' and consequent caregiving than neighbourhood or community.

Cheap labour perhaps, with unpaid kin, poorly paid servants and unpaid slaves as caregivers. If every caregiver had to be paid, there would have been major economic consequences. Children were necessary for survival and as helpers, and of course women.

Were there emotions attached? From epigraphic evidence it seems that individuals and families were praised and affection demonstrated. The catacomb inscriptions are unmistakably emotional, but whether they were they carved with due regard to public appearance or to express personal feelings is a little hard to say.

What did these inscriptions say about 'the family'? Frescoes tell us something, and in the Catacomb of Via Latina, the fresco is that of Hercules bringing the heroic Alcestis back from Hades to her husband

[1] Finally, let us keep care and caregiving in mind, for old and young, and give what is needed to help and care.

Admetus for whom she had sacrificed her life. Caring? Affection? Sceptics could suggest that such emotions may be for outward appearances rather than genuine affection. But the story of Alcestis and Admetus reads well of affection and sacrifice. Well worth a look-see.

y:

And from Philip Harland (2002) comes the caring:

For the two purest ones who also had faith in God:

> Marcus Demetrianos, who served as foremost archon, civic administrator, and director of contests with honor, and the dearest mother, Aurelia Pannychas. Aurelia Demetriane, their daughter, and Domitios Heliodoros, their son-in-law, together with her brother Demetrianos and her uncle Chrysippos erected this tomb as a memorial

Further emotional scenes are depicted in the loculus (long horizontal cavity in a catacomb) of Heliodora who was an adopted girl, and wanted to be in the company of her adopted father. It says, 'This is the tomb of Heliodora Pascasia whose foster-father died on the…of August…aged years…' (the ellipses mark missing information). The significance of this lies in the general knowledge that Romans deposited unwanted children outdoors to die, or be adopted or enslaved. So the fact of Heliodora wanting to lie in the company of her adopted father suggests considerable affection, for rescue from death and presumably a good life.

And the praise inscribed on the tombstones may not necessarily indicate good care in life, but it can point to a wish to record and show the virtues of the loved one.

Epitaphs can tell us of families where the values of human warmth, benevolence, tenderness, serenity and peace were in great honour.

Care and Spatiality—Where

So with kin, either born or adopted, and household members as caregivers, what did they have to do? The labour of caregiving brings us first to the spaces of caregiving, right into the heart of the practicalities of care.

We can split this space into different components, the first of which has emerged already in a discussion of kin, and servants and of home and household A second area is the space of the body which subdivides into the body itself, and also the space which that body does and can occupy, if it is mobile And that brings us into the wider community with the space possibly peopled with caregivers Fourthly, of less relevance here, is institutional space.

Within the household the space for and of care is doubtless the back rooms, the domain of women and of slaves, the domain of domesticity. In this space is the prime area of care, that of the body, and of the bed. Was this reachable by the infirm? Many beds were on platforms, or divans round the sides of the bedchambers, often in the 'retired' part of the house, according to 1 Kings. 22:25, Exodus 8:3, and Ecclesiastes 10:20, offering some form of privacy. There was maybe a mat or one or two quilts for covering. 1 Samuel 19:13 discusses bedclothes, though many people might sleep in the open air, wrapped in their outer garments. Pillows were of handy material, stones, seats, cushions, for example. However, for the most impoverished, beds were the bare ground, and covering was the outer garment.

Space in the beds themselves is interesting: were beds occupied by more than two or three in the family? If so, disability would therefore be visible, tangible, and likely to be assisted for example in turning, getting up or down. Or, of course, it could be annoying.

What would also be obvious were odours and noise.

Noise, in fact, could be a major issue in the houses, with ritual chants, prayers, and singing let alone the general noises of daily living, and perhaps noisy issues of ageing and some disabilities. In a small and very occupied space, the noise could perhaps be overpowering, at least to our ears. Would caregivers have to cope with the effects? Or would noise be a taken-for-granted situation?

Considerations of the space of the body itself show that cleanliness is important both in purification and for health, although the Muslims and Hindus castigated the early Christians for their uncleanness. At the same time, these early Christians objected to the preoccupation, and often licentiousness, involved with public bathing. Is it possible that the Christians' unhappy relationship with cleanliness is an example of their feelings about the body, asks Ashenberg (2007). And at the same time, in accordance with the inner purity of baptism, no one needed to bathe, as historian Virginia Smith says (2007). Although, it must be said, Matthew 6:17 talks of cleanliness in public, as 'when fasting, put oil on your head and wash your face, so that no one knows that you are fasting, but only the Father'. But presumably caregivers would maintain some form of bodily cleanliness, although hygiene for the sick and 'demonized' appears to be absent or limited. However, Acts 16:33 refers to the cleansing of wounds of Paul and Silas by their jailer. Whether the injured generally received such attention is in question.

But there's more to hygiene than bodily care. What happened to excess waste, when the disabled elderly were incontinent of urine and faeces?

Human waste for those unable to reach the privies was by perching or aiming into terracotta glazed pots, glazed to avoid odoriferous problems. The pots were then emptied into the privies.

Possibly the elderly sick unable even to use chamber pots might have worn some protection, later called 'winders' (German) for napkins. Washing was limited. Before or after using the latrine or chamber pot, there was no hand washing and food waste on hands was wiped by napkins. And since food was always eaten by hand, fingers always had to be wiped.

That meant more work for caregivers, whoever they were. Keep fingers wiped, keep napkins clean, I should imagine.

This presupposes a middle to wealthy household. What happened with the poorer people? Check out, through Martha Carlin's website, her discussion of St Radegund, from details by her biographer Fortunatus living in the sixth century AD who washed and scrubbed the bodies and heads of the paupers and the most needy. She plucked off worms, and dealt with scabs, lice and pus. When women 'descended into the tub, she washed their limbs with soap from head to foot.'

How many followed Radegund's lead and assisted the poor and needy, especially the elderly? There seems to be little if anything in the sources, nor much from the researchers in this area. So we could infer that poverty-stricken early Christians were dirty, had lice, and struggled with health problems.

A final aspect from this discussion is the sense of touch. The ideas that 'care' means 'touch', in feeding, helping with movement, probably toileting and bathing, could be supported by some of Robin Dunbar's (1996) comments in his work in *Grooming and Gossip and the Evolution of Language*. In his first chapter on p. 1, he calls attention to touch: 'A light touch, a gentle caress can convey all the meanings in the world: ....a calming influence, a declaration that intentions are friendly.... all social life is distilled in a single gesture'.

We could rephrase that with reference to caregiving: all care/affection/support is distilled in a single gesture. Is this overstating a possible descriptor of caregiving? Or can we infer, from our own knowledge, that such affection can exist?

And would such touch exist in these early days?
Why not?

Care—Groups

Additional to those receiving care at home with a loving and comfortable care, there were other individuals not comfortably at home. If we move outside the home into the streets, temples, and the old age homes, the chronically ill and disabled, some of whom were the elderly, were visible. Those without care and protection of family and household were to be seen everywhere in streets, baths, and forums, many homeless and begging.

This is where we see care working in the community. Can you imagine individual situations? Sick, with a rising temperature, cold or too hot, hungry, thirsty, mobile, non-mobile—and there's no one there? So you're out on your own in the areas of the city where few people venture at night. Here come some lay care members to help you!

Care by groups in the community is one of the highlights of Christianity which, at least in the first two centuries, was the only organization in the Roman world to give systematic care to the destitute sick. Such care was given by unskilled ordinary people in Church-based groups. Further on in history we have other groups focusing on those who needed care, and if we consider all these groups, we are emphasizing the work of different volunteers in a special work, that of caring for the plague victims some of whom would undoubtedly be elderly. And something to note is that not all the victims would necessarily be citizens but would still receive care. A needy person belongs to God, despite his religious beliefs and citizenship, according to John Chrysostom. The person was important, a distinction made by Christian philanthropy, says Timothy Miller (1997 p. 72) who refers to John Chrysostom and his 'new polis' which insisted on this distinction.

The major contribution of Christianity to care, then, is that the spirituality of the Christian message will result in major care of anybody in need. This, of course will include those elderly who were thrust from their homes if they were suffering from any of the serious epidemics of the times, such as leprosy, which would render them untouchable. These people were remarkably visible in the streets, as was the care given them. And this help came from individuals in the lay orders, those men and women who wished to belong to a religious order and to practise the religious life, but not to live in religious communities.

Christianity began a series of these lay movements, and the significance of many of these was that they performed the activities which would usually be done by members of the lowest classes. There are of course many more aspects to the groups than can be discussed here; they are a fascinating study within the culture of early Christianity. But that's a sideline. What is highlighted here is that they cared for people who needed help and had none. And although I step aside from the focus on elderly, it's worth doing so to take a closer look at these groups. They show the influence of Christianity on the development of caregiving which is offered to anyone in need, demonstrating a belief in the worth of all individuals who bore God's image. We turn back to St John Chrysostom and to the Christian concept of agape, the visible hallmark of social responsibility, moving us on from classical times.

Spoudaioi 4th–Seventh Centuries AD

Take the spoudaioi for example. It didn't seem that the spoudaioi were trained to care for the sick in any way, or that they were a nursing order. Various references say clearly that these members had no medical training. What they did was what would usually be performed by members of the lowest classes, the hands-on, mundane work, such as bodily and hygiene care.

These spoudaioi were volunteers, with some support from Church funds, or their own labour. It sounds as if these volunteers were the unemployed, and the help they could give was their 'daytime job'. Some were employed and supported themselves by their own labour, others were voluntary. The membership tended to be from the lower classes, but could include members of the aristocracy who wanted to dedicate themselves to service to God and the relief of suffering. Middle- and some upper-income men and women entered the order.

So this lay caring order represented a wider variety of social backgrounds than other movements, such as the decani and parabalani, who were very much drawn from the lowest classes.

While that doesn't necessarily affect the type of assistance given, what it does suggest is that the perception of the elderly, and disability, illness, and hurts, is not necessarily one of demonic views so that a cleric is needed, nor are the problems of such a taboo nature, of dirt and uncleanness, that these problems should only be managed by lower orders. In fact, it seemed that Christianity considered illnesses, infirmities, and bad health generally to be of natural causes.

The spoudaioi, and decani and parabalani (which latter two developed a 'guild-like status' and whose members were paid it seems), just gave the kind of assistance to the sick which lay people could perform. Community is often where the early Church's care of the sick took place. And why not? If there is a need for justification, Rabbi Joshua ben Levi from the early third century said that if the Messiah could treat the sores of all the lepers who lived outside the city gates, then taking care of other sick people should not be below the dignity of ordinary Jews. As Ferngren and others say, anyone who was poor and destitute, who lacked any relatives to care, would be left to rot in the streets. These were the people who the spoudaioi cared for.

There were other groups of such helpers: the philoponoi, the parabalani and the almanah, all of whom originated in the third century AD. The details of these groups give us some idea of who they were and what they did. Whether they were directly influenced by Christianity and the Christian message is not clear, but it seems a likely influence.

Philoponoi—3–Fourth Centuries AD

The philoponoi in Alexandria were a group of poor citizens, who dedicated their lives to helping others, and had close connections with local churches and monasteries. Like the ***parabolani***, the ***philoponoi*** were themselves indigent citizens who dedicated their lives to helping others. They were organized in groups, each with its space, linked with a hospital-area in a monastery where the***y*** would meet and possibly offer medical services.

Parabalani Third Century…

Another group is the parabalani or parabolanoi, the name of a medical corps meaning, in ancient Greek or Latin, 'those who risk their lives as nurses' or who disregard their lives to care for the sick and dying and to bury the dead. Like the philoponoi, they apparently came from the lower poorer classes of Alexandria, forming a corps to aid the sick. This could mean that the group originated in a time of plague, during which time these men risked extraordinary exposure to contagion. Eusebius talks of other people, whether voluntary or employed we don't know, who joined this group. Their fanaticism apparently caused sufficient problems that the authorities refused to allow more than 500 to be enrolled.

However, their strength was such that they were used as 'ambulanciers' who could carry lepers, for example, to leprosariums. They have been described as a 'company of ambulance men' or even paramedics.

Getting people off the streets to a safer place for care and treatment is certainly a major caring act.

Almanah—Third Century

The charitable care work was not confined to men, though. We come to the Almanah, the Order of Widows, a lay group of women.

It's worth considering the existence of the almanah in some detail. The existence of this group, considered as religious or semi-religious, challenges the rules for women. The root word, *alem*, for *almanah* [widow] meant 'unable to speak' and the women were dependent on male relatives to speak on their behalf. A brief reference here shows how revolutionary was this group: women in biblical Judaism and in many other of the Near Eastern societies at that time, were unable/not allowed to speak for themselves. Adult women had a social status determined by being a wife, mother, and mistress of the household. Being widowed therefore could mean considerable upheaval. Widows were to be supported by her sons if she had any; if none, her father-in-law should he still be around was expected to arrange another marriage for her. A widow who can't remarry and who has no sons is in a shaky position—she is truly 'unable to speak' and has no means of support. Sometimes she was forced into slavery or prostitution to survive. She could be socially ostracised and pushed to the edge of the kinship structure' as M. Cathleen Kaveny (2005) notes.

Though socially ostracised and ignored by the wealthy and powerful, biblical laws tried to ensure widows had some protection. Old Testament prophets objected to the oppression and in Israel the king was responsible to safeguard widows and other vulnerable groups. Nonetheless, the problem was there for many women.

However, having familiarised ourselves with the position of women, we might now have a look at the pragmatic details of these almanah members.

Historians have emphasized that women were significant in building and sustaining the Church, and many of these were powerful women, such as Phoebe, who protected Paul, or Lydia, the merchant of purple goods, and patroness of the apostles (Acts 16:14ff) for example. At the same time, and here we come to the nub of the matter, is that the early Christians were serious in their obligations to support vulnerable people in their midst, and these would include many of these widows. Apparently the Church at Rome was caring for 1500 widows and other poor persons. Some of these might well have been members of this Order.

Now we can begin to see what the Almanah, or the Order of Widows, was about. This was where the Church recognized the contribution that wealthy widows could make to the well-being and spiritual growth of their fellow believers. When discussing this, everyone refers first to Timothy who lists qualifications for membership of this Order. '60 years of age: only one marriage, and a history of good deeds. Only these could 'enrol' or be 'appointed' to the Order of Widows.'

Their first duty was to pray, obviously a care duty basic to thinking about others. But in other care terms, they visited to comfort, to fast, to pray with the sick and also to give practical instruction to younger women.

Writers say that this Order had as its focus a communal relationship with other like-minded women, maybe an innovative form at that time of social unity. Members were asked to inter-relate and consider contributing help, a set of activities which asks for more than a willingness to give alms.

The intrinsic meaning of this group is that older women contributed their spirituality to care and teach, to minister in this way to those in need: praying with the sick, teaching them, ceaseless prayer on behalf of the community and visiting the sick, especially sick women. It is unlikely that there was hands-on care, but there might have been an ensuring of sufficient care, an oversight, maybe a checking of food intake, bed linen, and perhaps suitable clothing. And certainly there would be advice to younger women involved in the household of the elderly.

This is certainly part of caregiving. It is often older women who visited the sick and elderly homebound, as well as practising the other bodily works of mercy. And it is older women who often cleaned the very Church building itself. In many ways, then, to rehabilitate the Order of Widows would simply be to give a name and formal recognition to the significant ministry that widows and elderly women already contribute to the Church.

Caregiving in these groups has a two-way benefit, it seems, because with the creation of a group such as the parabaleni or the almanah, the

Church recognised the need for involvement and direction and, particularly with women, it recognized the difficulties such women faced, socially and economically. Through the various Orders, it seems that the Church itself provided significant recognition and material assistance for the most vulnerable members of the community who had already given service to the community. The essence is spirituality, and the action is pragmatic.

So from here spirituality needs to be recognized very clearly and inserted into the vocabulary of caregiving, with its meanings of beyond the practical, non-material, things of the spirit, relating to religious belief. One dictionary offers 'spiritual home' in the sense of a feeling of 'belonging'. Perhaps this is what the almanah did for those who were sick and disabled, made them feel that they 'belonged' to the Christian sect, as it was then. There is permeating through the disability historical chronicles a sense of marginality, of being on the edge of society, of being unable to participate fully. What applies to the sick and disabled could also apply to their caregivers. Note, I'm using the word 'could' because who knows what other roles some of these caregivers occupied. However, the almanah, unable to 'speak' and unprotected by a near male relative, were definitely peripheral. Like unto like, perhaps.

References

Ashenberg, K. 2007. *The Dirt on Clean: An Unsanitized History*. Knopf.

Balch, David L. and Carolyn Osiek. 2003. Early Christian Families in Context, Wm. B. Eerdmans-Lightning Source.

Basil of Caeserea, What Answer Will You Make to the Judge? Sermon to the Rich, Article 13, Christian History Institute.

Biblical references are taken from the Holy Bible, English Standard Version

Carlin, Martha. 2004. Fortunatus and St Radegund, https://web.archive.org/web/20160412044654/http://mw.mcmaster.ca/scriptorium/radegund.html.

Christian History Magazine, Issue 101, (2011) Healthcare and Hospitals.

Dunbar, R. 1996. *Grooming and Gossip and the Evolution of Language*. Cambridge: Harvard University Press.

Epistle of Mathetes to Diognetus, Church Fathers, New Advent, Ch.5, https://www.newadvent.org/fathers/0101.htm.

Eusebius. 1926. *Ecclesiastical History, Volume I: Books 1–5*. Translated by Kirsopp Lake. Loeb Classical Library 153. Cambridge, MA: Harvard University Press.

Ferngren, Gary. 2007. *Medicine and Health Care in Early Christianity*. Baltimore: John Hopkins University Press.

Garland, Robert. 2010. *The Eye of the Beholder: Deformity and Disability in the Graeco-Roman World*, 2nd edn. London: Bristol Classical Press.
Harland, Philip A. 2002. *Connections with Elites in the World of the Early Christians,* Ethnic Relations and Migration in the Ancient World, https://www.philipharland.com, publications.
Kaveny, M. Cathleen. 2005. The Order of Widows: what the Early Church can Teach Us About Older Women and Health Care. *Christian Bioethics* 11 (1): 11–34.
Miller, Timothy S. 1997. *The Birth of the Hospital in the Byzantine Empire.* Baltimore: John Hopkins University Press.
Barbara, M. 1980. *Number Our Days Touchstone/Simon & Schuster.*
Porterfield, A. 2005. *Healing in the History of Christianity.* Oxford: Oxford University Press.
Richmond, David A Biblical Perspective on Ageing and Older People. https://www.selwynfoundation.org.nz/media/2052/.pdf.
St John Chrysostom, Homily on Matthew, Homily 50 on Matthew. https://www.newadvent.org/fathers/200150.htm.
Smith, V. 2007. *Clean: A History of Personal Hygiene and Purity.* Oxford: Oxford University Press.
Tertullian, Apologeticum. https://www.tertullian.org/works/apologeticum.htm (Tombstone references)

Further Recommended Reading

Bachmann Mercedes L. Garcia Bachmann, Women at Work in the Deuteronomistic History. No. 4 in the series International Voices in Biblical Studies, 2013, Atlanta, Society of Biblical Literature.
Baruffa, Antonio. 1989. The Catacombs of Saint Colitis, History Archaeology Faith Editrice Elle di Ci.
Bowersock, Glen W. B. 2010. In Anabases, 12. pp. 45–54. December 2010.
Brown, P. 2012. *Through the Eye of a Needle: Wealth, the Fall of Rome, and the Making of Christianity in the West, 350–550 AD.* Princeton University Press.
Catholic Encyclopaedia. 1913. www.catholic.org/encyclopedia.
Christian History Magazine, No. 101 (2011) Healthcare and Hospitals.
Crislip, Andrew T. 2005. From Monastery to Hospital: Christian Monasticism and the Provision of Health Care in Late Antiquity University of Michigan Press.
De Rossi, Giovanni Battista in article in Catholic Encyclopaedia.
Ferngren, Gary. 2011. A New Era in Roman Healthcare. *Christian History Institute Magazine*, 101.

Horden, Peregrine and Richard Smith eds. 1998. *The Locus of Care: Families, Communities and Institutions and the Provision of Care in Antiquity*. Routledge, New York.

Loewenberg, Frank M. 2001. *From Charity to Social Justice: The Emergence of Communal Institutions for the Support of the Poor in Ancient Judaism*. Transaction Publishers, and New Jersey.

Lysaught, M.T. 2005. Practicing the Order of Widows: A new call for an Old Vocation. *Christian Bioethics, 11*(1), 51–68.

Mazzoleni, Danilo. 1999. writes of Inscriptions in Roman Catacombs in a pictorial history of The Christian Catacombs of Rome, pub. Schnell & Steiner in 1999.

Meeks, W.A. 1983. *The First Urban Christians: The social world of the Apostle Paul* (pp. 59–60). Yale University Press.

Panciera, Silvana. 2014. *The Beguines, Women in Search of Sanctity Within Freedom*. Amazon.com Services.

Rosenwein, B.H. 2006. *Emotional Communities in the early Middle Ages*. Cornell University Press.

Simons, Walter. 2001. Cities of Ladies, Beguine Communities in the 1981) Medieval Low Countries, University of Pennsylvania Press, Philadelphia. P.67.68.

CHAPTER 7

Soundings from Later Middle Ages to the Renaissance—Fifteenth to Eighteenth Century

Introduction

With the wider variety of written resources in mediaeval and Renaissance times, looking at these gives us a far better opportunity to see more clearly a detailed range of caregiving situations than has been possible so far. It's obvious that there is greater and more accessible recording of a social awareness and recognition not only of giving care itself, but also a recognition of the assistance given to informal caregivers such as neighbours. And there is also an increase in the legal and political awareness. While such an awareness may have existed before, now we have it more clearly noted. Much of this support will be familiar to us in our own times and exploring the environment of individual caregiving in the past will reveal the unchanging activities of the caregiver. Even though the environment is different, and there is other help at hand, the caregiving status and role remains remarkably unchanged.

The Ageing Identity

To provide a vivid picture of elderly during these times, I propose to start off with age numbers, then move to definitions and descriptions.

Best estimate statistics of the elderly from the sixteenth to the eighteenth century suggest that the proportion of the population over sixty was 10%, falling to eight per cent by the end of the eighteenth century

B. Hale, *Historical Reflections on Care in the Western World*, https://doi.org/10.1007/978-3-031-87128-3_7

(Wrigley and Schofield 1981). Ageing as defined in the legislative documents is seen through the granting of age-linked exemptions from military service, trial by battle, service on the town watches, and various other public duties such as payment of taxes or obligatory work. These exemptions were granted to those of 60 or 70 years of age. In various other such texts, 60 is the indicator of old age. And despite the downturn in the ageing population, an aptly named book by Susannah Ottaway (2004), *The Decline of Life* states, 'there were enough old people to allow for mockery and satire as well as respect and care', a sentence which has been quoted by Ottaway in other books.

As well as numbers, age definition can depend on the ability to be productive, especially for the more impoverished elderly. It can also depend on the power of possessions. Lacking either of these, older people could be marginalised, linking them more with others of similar characteristics, those receiving 'pensions' and 'poor law' assistance, for example. Other characteristics which push older people into marginality were the particular features of ageing such as visible problems. Physical problems of poor mobility and general frailty, and the mental feebleness of forgetfulness and impairment made such older people immediately recognizable and liable to taunts and 'mockery' by some, or 'respect and care' by others. So say the aforementioned writers and also Troyansky and Shahar (1993) in their discussion on the aged in the Middle Ages.

In this period, 'old age' became increasingly defined by chronology as state bureaucracies grew, becoming more evident in the eighteenth century. The suggestion is that older people 'began to be considered as a social constituency in their own right' when in 1684 the first civil service pension was allocated and the first civil servant received a pension at age sixty. This information came from civil service organization fact sheets (civilservant.org.uk), and more information on pensions is available from Pat Thane's insightful works.

However, as well as the demographic and chronological descriptions, there are useful descriptions of ageing to be found in medical/health information. The medics of the time continued to work with the 'theory of humours and many elderly, particularly the very old, 'underwent changes of psychosomatic significance, giving rise to childish qualities'.

Such 'childish qualities' also included bodily weakness and loss of control. Clearly, the elderly were not necessarily defined just by a number. Rather, people were also defined as old based on capacity, fitness, and appearance rather than simply passing an age/number/milestone. Above all, the definition included the capacity to perform the normal tasks of adult life, especially work, and much of this is discussed by the numerous researchers in ageing at this time.

There was, then, no productivity and thus no power for many older people. However, public opinion emphasized that older people were to be particularly valued and respected as repositories of wise counsel to the young, who, in return, cared for and protected them. Rightly, there is some considerable scepticism here, considering the 'satire' and 'mockery' which some older people received, and the enforced labour in workhouses even for an enfeebled population. And there were, as seen in Chapter Three, a few myths and legends pertaining to ageing and care which challenged this moral public opinion, with plenty more to be found.

Issues

'For the frail elderly of these times', we would recognise many of the disabilities from today, although they might have different names in different centuries. In Katalin Szende's work on mediaeval Hungarian towns she comments 'A study of old age in mediaevatowns in Hungary notes that there were no baptismal or death records before the end of the sixteenth century.' (p. 198), so, as she continues, it was difficult to identify older people. Still, the arrival of old age could be identified by physical signs and obvious disability. The 'lepre', the blynde, the dumbe and the deaf, the creple, the lame and the lunatic And how fortunate we are to have such sources as this Historic England's outline on the internet of health issues.

Maybe because of the sources or because of the amount of contemporary work focusing on the sources, we have a great deal of information on issues, diagnoses, and treatments. I turn first to Hippocrates (relevant from c.460–370 BCE) who subscribed to the humoral medical theory, where bodily cooling and drying occurred in old age. Most people from 60s onwards had problems with breathing and catarrh, and difficulty with micturition, probably not only problematic passing urine but also retaining it, though Hippocrates does not mention incontinence. He also mentions arthritis, nephritis, dizziness, apoplexy, itching, sleeplessness, watery discharge from bowels and eyes and nostrils, dullness of vision, glaucoma and hardness of hearing. Enough? But there's more.

Consider, too, the loss of a limb. How was the body then used and managed? Prosthetics? This form of dependence is another care aspect rarely mentioned in general works. But more of the prosthetics later, when we come to discuss body space.

What was also a major consideration was incontinence. In mediaeval times this was dealt with was by strapping on cups for men and inserting pessaries for women to assist the problem at least overnight. Not an unusual solution to the problem, as pessaries and male clamps were used from the time of ancient Egypt but certainly something for the caregiver to use, help with, or at least be aware of the possibilities. And there were other forms of treatment, such as surgery or drugs to strengthen the nerves and muscles in the urethra. Naturally, these are from the health professionals, but what might involve caregivers is the use of hydrotherapy, involving cold baths and douches. A fascinating subject since it takes us right to the basics of caregiving, of cleanliness and of ensuring the better functioning of the body and its presentation.

And yet another set of issues which include, among others, lifestyle diseases, infectious diseases pain, neurological diseases. From the writings of Bill Bryson (2021) focussing on this 'wobble of flesh' on the first page, there appears a list of health problems deriving from mouse droppings. Bryson also mentions surgical procedures and their aftercare required.

So that's quite a list. With the addition of mental and cognitive impairments, and forgetfulness this gives us some idea of what the caregiver had to deal with.

Care—The Start

The caregiving context, as we know, begins with one person's need and another person's ability, willingness or duty-bound to meet that need. And a brief glance at caregiving in historical times not only shows glimpses of the close physical relationship of hands-on care but also the emotional, the powerful, and the burden/spiritual uplift which can exist.

And when we take a closer look at this one-on-one situation, we can also perceive the involvement of a variety of other people during this often lengthy process of caregiving at home. Appearing and disappearing individuals represent numerous systems with different capabilities of helping, and these specialists may form either ongoing or maybe intermittent relationships or become involved in a one-off advisory position. Much as they do today.

Spirituality is one of these, since, in the Middle Ages sickness was often seen as the result of heavenly intervention, and prayer was essential for healing. Medical intervention is another. Doctors were inspired by the Hippocratic theories of the ancient Greeks (approved by the Church) that four 'humors' in humans reflect the four basic elements of the world: blood, yellow bile, black bile and phlegm. Black bile or melancholy was particularly associated with earth, dryness, cold, autumn, and old age.

As in previous eras, these four humors must be balanced for an individual to remain healthy. The diagnostic task of the physician was to determine, by observing the patient, what humor had taken over. Fever in the patient indicated that the problem was one of yellow bile, while coolness and perspiration pointed to phlegm. In any event, bleeding, by opening a vein or applying leeches, was a method widely used to balance the humors. Some physicians preferred administering hellebore, a plant with harmful toxins. Such treatment provoked violent diarrhoea and vomiting and by this was supposed to remove the troublesome humor.

Another form of treatment which brings others into the dyad of caregiving, is that of help sought from wise women. One such was Mary of Eldersfield (b.1454), known by some as a witch and famous for her knowledge of herbal medicine, who used leaves of 'danewort' or the dwarf elder, to rub on a sprained knee, thus allowing the victim, Lord Edward of March, to mount his horse (Historic England).

Potions and spells can be considered just as much of an attempt to balance and control a sickness or disability as medicine, administered by the healer or maybe by the caregiver. Women at home were the first to be called on for medical care. For one thing they were cheaper. Then, if home remedies had been tried and failed, the work of local wise women would be called on. Care consisted of bandaging, healing mixtures to calm, or soothe inflammations. Wise women would concoct medicines, such as potions to be drunk or used to bathe the injury or inflammation, or smooth on as lotions or salves. These would be accompanied by a chant or prayer over the patient, and there was generally a limited or no charge.

There was, of course, no cure for ageing itself, but these home remedies might well be palliative treatments caring for anything ailing the older person.

Legal and Financial Care

Two other closely related systems involved with care, demonstrating that a form of care existed outside the immediate dyad, are those of the legal and financial means of support, involving individuals in the making of wills, and demonstrating a sense of power as well as reciprocity.

Some supports were obviously designed for the impoverished in the community—parish support payments; family support; and neighbourhood care and support, for those living alone—to ensure safe living at home. Reading Marjorie McIntosh's (2013) description of Hadleigh in Essex tells us much of what was organised by town officials to ensure elderly well-being. This is so interesting that I want to quote a paragraph or two:

> An overview of the town's role in providing relief suggests the scope of its system. Between 1579 and the early 1590s, an average of ninety-two people received help from the town each year, with an average payment of 18s.11d. annually; ... By the later 1590s, Hadleigh was spending as much as L180 annually on 120 to 130 needy people. Some of the assistance went to people living in their own homes who were essentially self-sufficient: they received aid merely in the form of occasional grants of goods or cash. Others were supported when sick or if their families could not provide a decent burial.... For those adults temporarily unable to look after themselves due to illness or injury the town paid for boarding with another family; (pp. 76, 77).

Family care and support for the poor depended on available resources. Robisheaux (1989) refers to Barbara Ziegler from Bachlingen in Southwest Germany in 1620. 'I stayed with my son for four years but the food was bad and he supported me with great effort' (p. 162). She is only one of many examples which Robisheaux reports.

Another form of support, this time for the wealthy, was negotiation for care whereby the farm or estate would be given to an adult child in exchange for specific provisions (Zuijderdujin and Overlaet 2021). Such support or care focused first of all on the space of the elderly. They could be housed in the younger family's home, with the use of a room, and rights to a certain amount of food, or the family could live in the house of the older person. Specific details of bed-and-board contracts appear in some of the documents: use of chair by fireside, use of latrine, use of scullery. Legally this was documented, handing over the 'messuage' of the land and house to older sons and wives.

Inheritance thus meant that care would be given, but what did that mean for the older person? In some countries, according to Horden and

Smith (2013) it meant that authority was transmitted to the next generation. The old person would 'retire'. The younger generation would assume the responsibilities for the estate, and for the older person's care. This could lead either to comfort within the familial home, or it could lead to considerable neglect and abuse as these authors above have emphasized.

But there was oversight of the contracts, so that if care broke down, then the inheritance could be withdrawn, the 'messuage' and the house could be taken away from the potential heirs.

Another system of support for frail older people was that the heir could pay for care, or there would be an annuity from which carers could be paid. This was a more popular option in northern Europe and one which allowed more freedom of choice of residence. presumably for the heir as well as the older person. The carers could be family members, paid for their work, distant relatives, or even hired nurses.

And yet snother example of financial arrangements comes from a sample of about 1,300 late mediaeval wills from three Hungarian towns, where 70 (6%) mentioned living parents, and individual testaments called for provision for an aged parent. This particular testament, dated November 1467, declared:

> I order that my father, Andre, has to be taken care of beside my son Wolfgang, and be provided with food and clothes as long as he lives in a proper way from my bequest. Should he, however, be impatient and unbearable because of his impatience, he has to be given a pension fund according to the council of the executors of my testament and of further honourable pensions...But I want that my father be taken care of in any case, as it was written above. (Troyansky, ibid.)

And more from Troyansky. Further wills and testaments demand the care of a mother-in-law, spelt out in her son's 1481 will in Pressburg:

> I leave to my wife that she should keep my mother with her and feed her as long as she lives, as I trust her [the wife]. Should it happen, however, that the two of them cannot stand each other, then I leave to my mother one of my vineyards named Perg by St Nicholas Church as long as she lives....

With these injunctions in the wills and testaments, there is no doubt that people felt responsible for those in need of care and that some sort of care would be available.

To recapitulate, the wealthy focused on inheritance patterns, and used servants to look after the needs of the body. The space in some homes which the ageing body occupies, the 'seat by the fire, the use of the latrine, place in the scullery, is far from the place of elderly in a struggling family where the wife may have to work in the fields and the shadow of the workhouse looms for those in need of constant care. Time for caregiving in these families is likely to be limited, so the elderly—probably leaky, certainly demanding—body might have to be moved because in economic terms for the caregiver, she might need to work or be forced to work. If she was deemed to be 'idle' she could be forced into employment. Being 'idle' included being under 60 years of age and not living by trade, nor exercising a particular craft, nor having assets… nor serving another. And this last does not appear to include giving care. The information comes from a 1349 ordinance noted by Judith Bennett (2010). If field work was not available or possible, there was other work for older women. They might be required as 'select women' to run schools in each parish (in Norwich in this instance, says Margaret Pelling (1991) to teach poor children how to spin and knit. And another job these women could do was to 'help neighbours at need' (p. 84) which seems an indeterminate role, but could include caregiving.

At the same time since it is highly likely that many women needed to work, and their caregiving duties, large or small, had to be provided by others. And these others might be by other kin, or neighbours.

There is considerable evidence of out-relief for elderly and the possibilities of their moving in and out of workhouses or age care institutions, when family care was unavailable, as it might well have been with women working in the fields at harvest time in particular. The topic of poor relief, parish out-relief, and the use of institutional care is large, and it proves that there was a major social need: and a religious conscience regarding care of the elderly, as noted in Pelling and Smith. And again to return to Marjory McIntosh, (2013) Hadleigh operated two types of residential institution for the needy: a workhouse and two almshouses in which thirty-two elderly people lived rent-free while receiving a weekly cash allowance plus firewood and occasional gifts of bedding or cloth.

How was this accomplished? McIntosh in her chapter (2) of Horden and Smith (2013) tells us that there was a combination of rental income from properties owned by the town, endowments for the poor, as well as current gifts and bequests distributed by the collectors, and local rates imposed on the wealthiest of the household heads.

Of interest here too is that though many of the elderly and poor had wealthier relatives nearby, there did not seem to be a requisition that families were solely responsible for their own poorer members.

Kin and Community Care

But the preference was always for family care. Older people stayed home when sick, as far as they could. Few wanted to be admitted to the workhouses of the era. so their support would be in their own homes, in the homes of their family members, or 'flatting' with other older people. Neighbourly care was also a likely case as well as kin.

Examples range from the simple to the more complex. Seventeenth-century Europe shows a variety of household structures. Bed-and-board contracts as we have seen, flatting and the general movement of family members contributed to a fluid household.

Care By the Community

Financially, the wealthy create care for themselves. Impoverished older people were supported by the parish, through the monies collected via the Poor Law in 1601, which could provide money to give support to the old and infirm. Pelling and Smith are exceptionally useful authors here as is Pat Thane, (1994). This might consist of money to purchase clothes, food or firewood—especially in hard winters. It might provide funds to cover medical expenses such as visits by a practitioner or to purchase specific remedies. In some cases, though, the parish might even pay people to actually move in and care for the elderly and infirm. In such cases, the elderly person had access to a relative level of care that many are assessed for today. The allotted person might cook and clean, perhaps administer medicines and, importantly, provide companionship. The gratitude of the recipients of this type of care is reflected in the fact that they often bequeathed what little they had to these (to use the modern term) 'carers', even if it was a few bedclothes or 'wearing apparel'. This level of care for that period is quite significant. Examples from different parish council records show as Pat Thane (2000) reveals:

- 1628 Mrs John Platt received between sixpence and a shilling weekly for caring for an aged bachelor neighbour. 'Goodwife Platt' was a carer, as was her husband. John Platt received six shillings per month for 'keeping Eldridge's boy' the child of a neighbour.

Alice Hall of Tonbridge which was a wealthy parish in Kent was widowed in 1789 and was entirely dependent on the community with no children to care for her. Care was a community effort. (Pat Thane, ibid.)
Alice Stock in Bishopsgate, London became aged and lame, she received 6d a fortnight to care for her 'foolish girle'.
If family care broke down, or parents died, then 'keepers ' or nurses in the local community would be paid to care for people. E.g. John Shusock of Wapping, London, was paid 2s 7d per week from 1649–53 to 'keep' the 'innocent' Thomas Walker, with extra payments for clothing and other necessaries. (https://historicengland.org.uk/research/inclusive-heritage/disability-history/1050-1485/)

Care was then not only by immediate kin but also by neighbours and friends. The town of Hadleigh in Essex had not only care by kin and help from the community but also there were no categories of distinction between public, private, formal and paid, and informal care.

Care, in fact, was a general role of support as further examples from seventeenth-century parishes show. Parishes considered that care was a fundamental need, and the parish council helped financially. The community supported the carer and ensured that care was delivered at home, if parental or family care ceased for any reason.

This would undoubtedly have maintained older people at home in some degree of comfort and safety, and also this spirit and will to care listed in parish records beyond the seventeenth century show concerns for younger people: caring for 'innocents' or 'fools' living with their families, and those with lameness, missing limbs, blindness, or deafness. Many of these younger people worked, married, usually to non-disabled people, and the marriages were apparently stable and long lasting. Those with learning disabilities as 'natural fools' and 'ideots' would live with families, and if families were struggling to cope financially because of ill health then parish relief could be paid. This shows care for the younger people and their caregivers. Were such services also forthcoming for the elderly? Yes and in a variety of ways.

One example is the petition presented no doubt to the Quarter Sessions in 1657 by Edward Fox in Nottinghamshire: 'his wife being very much distracted in her witts hath of late pulled down part of his dwelling house wherein she was kept, which by reason of his poverty he was not able to build up.' The court ordered that the house be rebuilt at the parish's expense, and the expectation was that the wife be maintained therein.

Further help in the community came from a lay group of women called the beguines who lived in a beguinage, or house for the beguines. Walter Simons (2001) has given a detailed account of these women who added to the group of potential carers in the community. This women's group, begun in the thirteenth century and mostly in the Low Countries was spiritually based, but non-monastic in that these women took no formal religious vows. They lived in voluntary poverty with their focus on care of the poor and sick.

The reason for the existence of the beguines is of less importance here than their focus. This was to help, to care, and be free to do so, through, among other activities, 'works of mercy' assisting old people, sick people in the infirmary or at home (particularly in case of contagious diseases, as in these cases hospitals do not accept sick people) and accompanying dying people One of the beguines, Ida of Nivelles (1197–1232) became a beggar to beg help for her companions, and with them she engages in nursing the sick. Three other short stories add to the picture:

Margaret of Ypres[1] begged also and Marie of Oignies (1177–1213) married at age 14 and she and her husband adopted the ideal of voluntary poverty, and dedicated themselves to the cure of lepers in a nearby infirmary for 12–15 years. Whether they themselves actually cared by helping the lepers or whether they gave money to those who did is not clear. The lepers were explicitly rejected from society, but thanks to these women, they were cared for, as Simons (2001) has noted.

Begging help for companions and then providing care now enters the vocabulary of care: as does working with the hands, to feed those in need outside, as well as the beguine companions inside the beguinage.

Unlike the previously described lay orders, the beguinage did form themselves into a type of institution; there were beguine houses, institutionalized maybe as were the convents. From these institutions, women

[1] xxx.

went to work as caregivers, according to Simons (ibid.) for single, women and their children. And various authors describe the beguines as working with lepers as well. Their work not only suggests a focus on the mundane as well as the spiritual, but caregiving for those in need, and this could surely extend to the unwanted elderly. In fact, the beguinage at Douai, of 18 beguinage movements during 1280–1360, focused on the poor and elderly in their community as MaryAnne Gonzales (2021) has written.

'Extending their work as carers and nurses, and also because their prayers were held in high regard—and that is worthy of note in the spirituality of care—the beguines were often asked to help those dying, to lay out the body and conduct the wakes, and also accompany the dead to their grave.'

Could this also be a form of caring? Why not? Spiritually, the dead move to another world, and therefore care on that journey is required, staying with the dying, and the dead until the body was buried, and 'keeping watch'.

From Outside to Inside—HOME

From the extensiveness of care outside the home by those in the community I want to change perspective and look closely at the minutiae of caregiving, beginning with the space of the body, then considering where it is housed, and how far it can move.

Any assessment of space in these times will extend beyond the body to particular areas of caregiving: bed place—on the floor, against the wall, movable, or immovable; the possibility of a number of occupants, mattresses and coverings, and maybe special equipment. Include in this assessment a survey of the general household hygiene, the furniture and cooking equipment. And then we can focus on how these spaces were used, what was in the house or household, including furniture. Within spatiality, we also have temporality, the length of time daily, perhaps, required for caregiving, and the length of time for care until death.

Looking and thinking about caregiving space develop ideas about intangibles such as familiarity and spatial distance, and, particularly from our contemporary experience, privacy.

Familiarity goes beyond the people concerned to a close knowledge of particular pieces of furniture: bed and mattress; special chairs perhaps; special equipment or clothing for the incontinent? Distance involves considering the amount of space between useable furniture, areas, doors, steps, for example, and calculating the possibilities of moving between these. And among these considerations the notion of privacy might be introduced, maybe as a limited concept in these early years.

Privacy may be a limited concept in these early centuries, with early recognition of the concept in different situations, according to David Vincent (2016). However when in the later Middle Ages and Renaissance times, the growth of more and larger houses between the castles and cottage levels, there is a sense of a growing taste for privacy where the chamber expands its usage to become more of a private parlour.

Imagine ourselves back in these mediaeval times, and being admitted to someone's home. What would we see first? If it was the home of the poorest people, we would most likely see floors first as we open the door into the living and often bedroom, as we now would designate a room holding a bed or bedding. For the poor, the top layer of rushes and straw on the floor was removed at times, leaving the bottom layer as a mass of filth and undoubtedly housing mice, rats, bugs, all of which would find their way into the home itself. For the needy cared-for individual, lice were probably constant companions, as indeed they were for many people. And caregivers no doubt had to deal with them. But other bugs and rodents might have caused other difficulties, dirt in particular, to infiltrate the home, and compound the problems of hygiene and infections.

In a number of houses there were beds attached to the wall that would have had to be folded out each evening.

Then, important in caregiving too, we have the mattresses. In the fourteenth century, we are looking at feathers for bedding, straw and litter too, and even, believe it, 'One description for which I cannot find the reference is still so telling that I want to include it. I would have you know that the mattresses on which I rest my limbs are stuffed with nothing but the moustaches of those my sword has vanquished.'

Straw however, remains the major filling for mattresses. For those in the upper echelons, bed-making was of loose straw, with a yeoman of the chamber rolling up and down on it to make it smooth and no daggers hidden in it. Then a canvas was laid over the straw, then the featherbed, smoothed with a bed-staff. And next, we have the coverings, 'fustians' or blankets and linen, all perfumed. Over all is a 'pane' of ermine. Or there might be a luxurious featherbed.

Needless to say this equipment is only found among the wealthy. Otherwise we find plain straw for mattresses which were covered, or cloths, stuffed with straw, laid on the floor against the wall, pulled up every morning to ensure more space.

In the small rooms of the poor there was usually only one bed. So what happened?

Sharing the bed or as Ekirch (2006) puts it, 'bed etiquette' meant that the children and women went to the back, while men slept at the front, since they were the ones to finish locking up the house. And there were chamber pots nearby for the women only and in Ekirch's vivid portrayal of night-times then, he describes how women of the house would fight over the one chamber pot. Men peed in the ashes of the fireplace.

What happened if and when the straw was wet or soiled? Was it left to dry out, shaken clean, or what happened to it? Replacing it would be costly.

Continence products would also be costly, but useful. For those who could afford it, equipment to deal with incontinence was usually a belt strapped to a bag. The bag was made either of animal skins or often leaves were used, and apparently milkweed leaves were the softest. Outside, of course, there were no problems, as the great Pepys maintained: he describes how his wife 'did her business' in the gutter. For women, there were napkins or pessaries.

There was much that carers needed to know. For example, the use of brimstone to help nightly cramps, as Parson Woodforde (late eighteenth century) did, holding it near the affected parts, with immediate beneficial results. Or a roast mouse, as a remedy for bed-wetting, was upheld by one mother writing to endorse its efficacy.

Further treatment for rheumatism (or cramp, some say) a bag of corks between the sheets or under the mattress helped to allay the pains. Another useful piece of knowledge was how to prevent bedsores. Two buckets of fresh spring water under the bed every day. Obviously this could only be done where there was available fresh spring water. Further knowledge for the caregivers was to insist that they never used cold boiled water because this apparently angered the Devil.

And further care knowledge is still of magic. Well within the context of caregiving is the following: smooth the hollow in the bedclothes to prevent the shape of the sleeping body being attacked and injured by sticking sharp objects into that shape.

Bed space, its layers, its comfort and its usage is definitely part of the caring context and part of which we might see as we first enter home space.

What else was within the caring context? Much of caregiving would depend on sensory awareness,

The smells would have been unpleasant, to our nostrils. But as St Bernard says where all stink, no one smells, quotes Ashenberg (2008) in her first chapter (ibid.). With so much information on the environment, as well as the disabilities occupying that environment, we could begin to consider the need and use the senses in giving care: touch, hearing, smell, and sight. And for many of the elderly, caregiver touch would have been of considerable importance. Touch involves the perceptions of pressure and of pain, of heat and cold. And the inner sense of feeling say, pain, hunger, thirst, need to empty the bladder, is also present. These sensations and perceptions are sensitised into caregiving too. Awareness of pain, of heat and cold and pressure is important. Gentle and helpful, sensitive or rough, pushing and possibly deliberately abusive. The touch of the caregiver in caring for the elderly and disabled body is extremely important. But we seem to have no indications of this. A read through of Parson Woodforde or Pepys's diary might give some indication.

Likewise the senses of hearing and of smell: hearing the feelings and wishes, and interpreting the sounds; and smell, of something perhaps out of the usual array of odours. Sight is also important in all caregiving and at all times. To see and then analyse the condition of the older person is important in caregiving. And to deal with the issues, observe, and respond requires major expertise also. These senses indicate some degree of familiarity within closely shared environments concerning tending the body, its needs and its movements.

So caregiving should stand tall with other health professions and become as visible as they are.

Such bodily needs require the ability and authority of other people in meeting such needs and when this failed and still fails to happen, then different authorities were called in to deal with possible abuse situations. These authorities were the local legal representatives, or the local parish council welfare representatives.

How public or hidden were the problems of caregiving and elderly? For 'lunatics', the spatial element is vital in the family's view, with the 'lunatic' being hidden as far as possible in a separate living space. Maybe this also took place for society's elderly, living at home. If there was no possibility of hiding or tucking the invalid into a back room, this would have brought the family's problem into the public arena, although given the closeness of living quarters, and busyness of the streets, it seems unlikely that there could be any such secret. By keeping the elderly family member or the family 'lunatic' more visible, it meant they were participating in family life as fully as they could.

If a move had to be made, then the question was where to? Moving from family and home, to community in a lodging contract, or to institutional care and treatment could infer a hierarchy of care responding to increasing need and inability of the family to cope, or the needs of the family to be earning. The questions are: who decided? And on what basis? And how was the movement accomplished?

Places to move to were hospitals, often church or monastery-based, poorhouses, initiated and supported by communities, and workhouses likewise.

But more of them later.

Bodily Care and Orthotics

So, back to the personal.

Closeness of people gave warmth and security. Privacy was an emerging idea, as Diana Webb (2007) discusses. Sleeping in one bed, with others, and in one room, does mean that help would be available if and when required. It also might mean that there was so much help that independence as well as privacy was a forlorn notion, and possibly a contemporary one. However to counteract dependence, the body could be balanced by artificial means, and I present some information on orthotics here. Balancing the body and bringing it back to the normal body posture brings in caregiving in the wider sense, with craftsmen thoroughly involved. And certainly there would be caregiving in the domestic sense to assist the fitting and use of orthotics. And I choose to add the craft of orthotics here into our notion of caregiving. Not, of course, in the intimate sense of bodily care but in the sense of maintaining balance and as much independence to the body as possible, and therefore lessening the need for care.

Many orthotics such as 'peg legs' could be fashioned by the peasantry themselves, while the more sophisticated orthotics, such as hands, would require considerable technical skill.

Generally, our knowledge of the Renaissance is that while it ushered in new perspectives of art, philosophy, science, and medicine, it expanded much further than that. By returning to the medical discoveries of the Greeks and Romans concerning prosthetics, the Renaissance also proved to be a rebirth in the history of prosthetics, beginning it seems with Ambroise Pare IV, according to Philippe Hernigou (2013b). These were generally made of iron, steel, copper, and wood, and it was common for tradesmen, including armourers, to design and create artificial limbs. People of all trades often contributed to making the devices; watchmakers were particularly instrumental in adding intricate internal functions with springs and gears.

Probably these carefully manufactured prostheses were only for the badly wounded wealthy. Nevertheless, it is interesting to see that to assist in returning the individual to a balanced whole person, such orthotics were made available. For example, in 1508, German mercenary Gotz von Berlichingen had a pair of technologically advanced iron hands made after he lost his right arm in the Battle of Landshut. The hands could be manipulated by setting them with the natural hand and moved by relaxing a series of releases and springs while being suspended with leather straps (Ashmore et al. 2019).

And around 1512, an Italian surgeon travelling in Asia recorded observations of a bilateral upper extremity amputee who was able to remove his hat, open his purse, and sign his name. Another story surfaced about a silver arm that was made for Admiral Barbarossa, who fought the Spaniards in Bougie, Algeria, for a Turkish sultan.

Further information comes from the mid- to late 1500s. French Army barber/surgeon Ambroise Paré has been thought of as the father of modern amputation surgery and prosthetic design. He introduced modern amputation procedures (1529) to the medical community and made prostheses (1536) for upper- and lower-extremity amputees. He also invented an above-knee device that was a kneeling peg leg and foot prosthesis that had a fixed position, adjustable harness, knee lock control and other engineering features that are used in today's devices. His work showed the first true understanding of how a prosthesis should function. A colleague of Paré's, Lorrain, a French locksmith, offered one of the most important contributions to the field when he used leather, paper and glue in place of heavy iron in making a prosthesis.

Noise

A final comment on the ageing and caregiving context links with the commentary on experiencing the living environment. Although rarely brought into the experiences of caregiving, the sensory aspect of hearing and noise have their places within the carerscape. Hearing, of course, in terms of deafness has always been a major consideration in caregiving, but noise is new, and had I not discovered David Hendy's work (2013) I doubt whether I would have given noise a thought.

But Hendy is enlightening and visionary in his work. His chapter on 'Shutting In' talks of the street noises of Edinburgh, among other things. He talks of noise being a 'jolt to the senses, with the first layer of noise in the streets, the 'chinking and clattering of pattens on the cobbles as people went about their business' (p. 171). Noise decreased as the evening wore on but the wearing of 'pattens' or wooden shoes and clattering on the cobbles or up and down the stairs, would have disturbed any sleeping caregiver or cared-for person. The noise during the day could be quite horrendous, with rumble and clatter of working people up and down the Mile, or High Street. However this diminished by eight o'clock when the 'great bell' was rung, to keep people in order. This was also the signal for the emptying of chamber pots and household wastes, accompanied by warning yells of GARDEZ LOO (p. 172).

Noise indoors of servants? Hendy (ibid) 2013) discusses this too (pp. 172ff). His main contribution to the care concept, however, is house noise, or just-outside house noise. He refers to Gladstone's Land and other tenements where the only access is via an outside staircase, which is always open. The soundscape at night of Edinburgh was full of terror. Everyone in a building shared a common staircase, and there were no separate servants' quarters in the building. Gladstone's Land like many of the other tenement houses was shared by people of different social strata, whose attitude to noise might differ. Privacy, our modern concept, was certainly not in existence at that time, although there might have been some wishing for it.

What this might have meant for caregiving we can only infer. Someone always around, perhaps, maybe able to help if necessary? Or perhaps a lack of solitude? Someone to disturb the rest both of the aged and of the carer? A relaxed feeling of knowing you were among people, neighbours who could probably be friends? It would depend on individual feelings and the individual experience.

In conclusion to this chapter as usual I want to draw up lines of visibility and language and to add the notion of balance, again, into the carerscape.

Visibility is apparent, as usual, legalistically. However, this does mean that care has been considered. Care is also inferred by the treatment of the medics. By providing the remedies, we can presume an aftercare. Neighbourliness, whether good or bad, is stated, as is parish welfare, and also it could be inferred by the architecture of the townhouses. This of course has happened before, in the household arrangements of early societies, and in the Christian lay movements. But here we can only infer that neighbours could help in the caregiving process.

Caregiving, then, has expanded into more detail of bodily and environmental space, and crowded with people, as seen from our contemporary notions of privacy and independence; also emphasized here are the sensory aspects of smell, which has appeared in other chapters, and of hearing and subsequently a brief comment on noise and how it could disturb the environment.

References

Ashenberg, Katherine. 2008. *The Dirt on Clean: An Unsanitised History*. Berkeley: North Point Press.

Ashmore, Kevin, Sergio Cialdella, Alberto Giuffrida, Elizaveta Kon, Maurillo Marcacci, and Berardo Di Matteo. 2019. Artifacts: Gottfried "Gotz" von Berlichingen- The "Iron Hand" of the Renaissance. *Clinical Orthopaedics and Related Research* 477 (9): 2002–2004.

Bennett, Judith M. 2010. Compulsory Service in Late Medieval England. *Past & Present* 209 (1): 7–51.

Bryson, Bill. 2021. *The Body: A Guide for Occupants*. New York: Anchor Books.

Ekirch, Roger. 2006. *At Day's Close: Night in Times Past*. New York: W. W. Norton.

Gonzales, MaryAnne. 2021. *Charitable Communities: Beguines and Charity in Later Medieval Douiai 1218–1360* (Doctoral Dissertation, University of Guelph).

Hendy, David. 2013. *Noise: A Human History of Sound and Listening*. London: Profile Books.

Hernigou, Philippe. 2013a. Ambroise Paré's life (1510–1590): Part I. *International Orthopaedics* 37 (3): 543–547.

Hernigou, Philippe. 2013b. Ambroise Paré IV: The Early History of Artificial Limbs (from Robotic to Prostheses). *International Orthopaedics* 37 (6): 1195–1197.

Historic England: Disability in the Medieval Period 1050–1485. (https://magic-spells-and-potions.com/herbs/herbal_simples.htm (re Mary of Eldersfield)

Historic England. https://historicengland.org.uk/research/inclusive-heritage/disability-history/1050-1485/

https://historicengland.org.uk/research/inclusive-heritage/disability-history/1485-1660/daily-life-of-people-with-disabilities/

https://www.attends.com/us/en/blog/history-of-urinary-incontinence-and-hygiene-pad-technology.html

Horden, Peregrine, and Richard Smith. 2013. *Locus of Care: Families, Communities, Institutions and the Provision of Welfare Since Antiquity*. London: Routledge.

Ottaway, Susannah. 2004. *The Decline of Life: Old Age in 18th Century England*. Cambridge: Cambridge University Press.

Mckintosh, Marjorie. 2013. *Poor Relief and Community i Hadleigh, Suffolk* 1547–1600. Univ. of Hertfordshire Press, paperback

Pelling, Margaret. 1991. *Life, Death and the Elderly: Historical Perspectives*. London: Routledge.

Pelling, Marga*ret* and Richard M. Smith (1994), eds, *Life,Death and the Elderly. Historical Perspectives*.Routledge, UK

Robisheaux, Thomas. 1989. *Rural Society and the Search for Order in Early Modern Germany*. Cambridge: Cambridge University Press.

Simons, Walter. 2001. *A City of Ladies: Beguine Communities in the Mediaeval Low Countries, 1200–1565*. Philadelphia: University of Pennsylvania Press.

Thane, Pat. 2000. *Old Age in English History: Past Experiences, Present Issues*. Oxford: Oxford University Press.

Troyansky, David, and Shulamith Shahar. 1993. Who Were the Old in the Middle Ages? *Social History of Medicine* 6 (3): 313–341.

Vincent, David. 2016. *Privacy: A Short History*. Cambridge: Polity Press.

Webb, Diana. 2007. *Privacy and Solitude in the Middle Ages*. London: Hambledon Continuum.

Withey, Dr Alun. Blog. https://dralun.wordpress.com/2012/03/30/caring-for-the-elderly-lessons-from-history-3/.

Wrigley, Edward Anthony, and Roger S. Schofield. 1981. In *Their Population History of England 1541–1871: A Reconstruction*. Edward Arnold Cambridge Group for the History of Population and Social Structure.

Zuijderdujin, Jacob, and Kim Overlaet. 2021. Strategies for Old Age and agency of the elderly in towns of the Low Countries in the Renaissance. *Continuity and Change* 26: 265–284.

Further Reading

Hale, Beatrice, Patrick Barrett, and Robin Gauld. 2010. *The Age of Supported Independence*. Dordrecht: Springer.

King, Helen. 1991. *Anthropology and Nursing*. London: Routledge.

Metzler, Irina. 2013. *A Social History of Disability in the Middle Ages: Cultural Considerations of Physical Impairment*. London: Routledge.

Panciera, Silvana. 2011. *The Beguines: Women in Search of Sanctity Within Freedom*. Gabrielli, San Pietro in Cariano (Verona).

Suzuki, A. 2013. Framing Psychiatric Subjectivity: Doctor, Patient and Record-Keeping at Bethlem in the Nineteenth Century. In *Insanity, Institutions and Society, 1800–1914*, 115–136. Taylor & Francis. https://doi.org/10.4324/9780203025789-14.

Wright, Lawrence. 1962. *Warm and Snug; the History of the Bed*. London: Routledge.

CHAPTER 8

Soundings from Eighteenth to Nineteenth Centuries

Introduction

Maybe we should designate the eighteenth century as the age of turmoil, a turbulent hundred years or so for many countries. During these hundred years, there were several wars in Britain and Europe. There were wars in India, and there was, of course, the American Revolution in 1775–83, diminishing British colonial power. Generally speaking, it was an exceptionally turbulent period of time for many countries. France and Spain, for example, were involved in the Seven Years' War (also called the French and Indian War) from 1756 to 63, and there were several wars with Spain such as the Anglo-Spanish War and the War of Jenkins' Ear while within Britain itself and earlier was the last rebellion of Scottish Jacobites, beginning in 1745 and ending at the Battle of Culloden in 1746.

Not only was there physical unrest, the eighteenth century saw major changes with the Industrial Revolution, and Scotland itself was particularly active. Along with the Jacobite Rebellion, there were notably the Highland Clearances, from mid-century to the middle of the nineteenth century. This period was also known as the Scottish Enlightenment, making it an intellectual powerhouse, with David Hume, Adam Smith, and Rabbie Burns. However, migrating first from their homes and then from their country was the central point of living for many. Details of the Industrial Revolution such as an increasing standardisation of hours

B. Hale, *Historical Reflections on Care in the Western World*,
https://doi.org/10.1007/978-3-031-87128-3_8

of work, the movement of people to find jobs, and increasing mechanisation all had an effect on bodies both younger and older. As Newman and Turner say in Chapter Seven of Craig-Atkins and Harvey (2024): 'The onset of old age was not simply determined by reaching a particular chronological milestone, but by class, occupation and gender.'

And as they also assert, the history of old age and that of disability are inextricably linked, because 'disablement was itself conceptualized as a form of ageing in working-class communities.'

And now to the stories of varying needs for warmth, shelter, food, for assistance to toilet, to dress, even to move, of protection from abuse, of poverty, these let us into a world at once familiar and unfamiliar.

But is there anything different in this century? Maybe its turbulence and the considerable movements which took place had some influence on care for the elderly. Movement to jobs could and did distance families from their elderly, and even when they were closer, the timing of work in the factories meant a non-attendance of kin caregivers. And there were the Clearances which meant large-scale movements.

At the same time bodily issues may indeed have changed or intensified, so what are the results?

Who then helped? Kin, neighbours, friends? When the elderly and indigent had no kin helpers, failed to find other helpers, what happened? When families had to move, did the elderly go too? Or stay behind? And then what happened?

Turn to the sources!

And so plentiful are the sources for this period of time that reading about ageing in eighteenth-century England is like combining a jigsaw of pieces of care. From individual care by kin to community at home and then to institutional or workhouse/poorhouse care we have a pattern of care showing how the elderly were looked after. Many diaries found and discussed (Ottaway 2004) show a series of varied relationships from care to abuse, financial support from the elderly to the young, and some of this returned generationally: as being from the younger to the older. The recording of friendship, of quarrels, of likes and dislikes create images of older and younger in a whirl of relationships and of care. In fact, Ottaway's detailed discussions from her large array of sources (which she has divided into primary and secondary) provides us with the information we want.

The array of detail makes for an exceptionally complex chapter, with considerable information on living at home with an illness/disability.

Information on kin and individuals when living at home was the ideal, but when there is no one there to provide care then the community provided parish relief and, importantly, institutions such as almshouses, workhouses, poorhouses—call them what you will, but places where indigent and disabled older people might find some form of care. Many of these are the result of the Elizabethan Poor Laws requiring support for elderly indigent and disabled, impoverished individuals. Some originate from religious houses. But there is no doubt: there they are, formal institutions with their role to shelter those in need, and with rules and regulations in place. Home care even without kin, was possible.

Ageing

Thanks to researchers such as Ottaway, Thane, and Newcome and Turner, we have what we could call an expanding view of 'the elderly'. Figures from Peter Laslett (1965) show less than 25% of the population of England to be over 40. But recent research from the above scholars has suggested that culturally the view was of bodily ability or disability rather than figures, dividing the population into younger and older, or fitter and disabled. These researchers talk in terms of older and the disabled having to struggle with a number of problems. As they say, there was no systematic welfare provision, and there were clearly difficulties in relying on kin, at least in some cases due to the turbulent times, especially as from these writers we learn that the main goal of the elderly as they age was to maintain independence until the end, and to help their families and the wider community for as long as they could.

But what happens when independence fades due to health problems? These historians write that older people in this period often turned both to family members and to the assistance available in many local communities, through informal sources of charity and importantly too, through the formal system of poor relief, which had existed in England since the foundation of the Elizabethan Poor Laws in the early seventeenth century. These were to ensure the welfare of the poor and disabled, and certainly included elderly disabled and indigent. The Poor Laws created an ability to meet needs by providing indoors sustenance and/or financial relief and by building and maintaining almshouses for those unable to live alone and with no relatives to assist.

So from care in the home by kin, friends, neighbours, we have care in the community in more formalised terms.

What were the needs? Failing health with a large category of problems, diminishing eyesight, and lameness all struck the elderly then, as they did before and just as they do today. And ageing, whether fit or less fit, does not always receive a sympathetic treatment. Devoney Looser (2005) comments on Frances Burney's *Evelina* (p. 34) which includes

> [...] a notorious scene of illegal betting on a foot-race between two old women. The women—chosen because they are older than 80 and strong—fall from over exertion, are plied with wine, and complain of injury. One ultimately slips and falls so badly that the other is declared the winner. A contemporary found that reading the account of the race "excited a roar of laughter" and a more recent critic called it one of the novel's "most delightful incidents." Other readers have expressed horror. Burney's good characters deplore the race....but the established pattern in Burney's fiction is one of using the pain faced by old women to provoke readers' laughter (Mrs Mirvan is another example). (p. 304)

Given, then, that there are various views of the elderly and ageing, what were the main issues?

Issues

Of course there were the various diseases, plague being just one, tuberculosis another. Other issues as well as bodily frailty are those of various diseases such as typhoid, scarlet fever, tuberculosis, cholera, and whooping cough.

Another list could start with war wounds and continue with the problems brought on by industrialisation. Oliver and Barnes (2012) among others have argued that industrialisation caused numerous problems. Factory production, mechanisation, standardised hours rather than working as able-bodied, weakened some of the workforce as many writers have said, for example, Gleeson (1999) and Kuskey (2016) to name just two. In fact, one vivid description by Kuskey (ibid.) is well worth quoting:

> Disproportionately short compared to the length of his arms and torso, and his non-functioning left index finger is displayed prominently against the brim of his hat. The illustration invites the reader into the book to discover what kind of life could have produced this body. In addition to telling his life story to Brown, a middle-class journalist who composed and published the Memoir for him, Blincoe testified before Parliament as to

> the long-term effects of factory work, displaying his deformities and scars as evidence authenticating the book's claims. (p. 4)

And in a study by Cambridge historian Ella Sbaraini (2021) looks at the suicides of older people in the eighteenth century. She takes evidence from 106 coroners' inquests which were uncovered in archives in London, Kent, Cumbria, Essex, Suffolk, and Bath. These records highlight the distressing issues facing older people in the 1700s—many of which remain major concerns today, including memory loss, loneliness, financial and occupational vulnerability and worrying about becoming a burden. She describes three older men, who suffered from fear of poverty, from loss of words/memories and with confusion.

But what constitutes 'disability' is closely connected to understandings of temporality, ageing and how a particular culture or society conceives of a normative life course, so says Ljuslinder and colleagues (2020, p. 26). Industrialisation changed the normative life course.

The complexities of disability from the Industrial Revolution seem to merge ageing into a description of people with disabilities so that the notion of ageing, vulnerabilities, and slowing down became confused with the general disabilities created by factory production. Physical debility had traditionally been seen as ushering in old age, but as industrialisation developed, concerns were increasingly raised that new modes of production were hastening physical decline making people 'old' before the customary 60 or 70 years (Ottaway, 2007, p. 17).

And disabilities required care with caregivers to deliver that care.

Care: Kin

The usual caregivers were kin and their duties were made clear.

Sources here range through a variety of documents, from the King James Bible, through literature, to archival material. And I begin with the societal rules, laid down in the Bible which most people would have heard, though not all would have read.

The duty to care was clear. Can we do better than take Romans 13:8–10, which commands 'love' in every verse. Job 12:12 insists that 'with old age comes wisdom, and with length of days understanding.' And in 1 Timothy 5:8: 'But if anyone does not provide for his relatives, and especially for members of his household, he has denied the faith and is worse than an unbeliever.' Leviticus 19:32 states, 'You shall stand up before the gray head and honor the face of an old man, and you shall fear your God: I am the Lord.' And Acts 20:35 says, 'In all things I have shown you that by working hard in this way we must help the weak and remember the words of the Lord Jesus, how he himself said, "It is more blessed to give than to receive".' And one more; Psalm 71:9: 'Do not cast me off in the time of old age; forsake me not when my strength is spent.'

These are the rules of life, laid down by universal religious texts. None of them say how care is to be delivered, for how long and how the hands-on, regular caregiver looks after herself—and it usually is a woman.

More evocative and of course less rule-conscious, is care seen through various works of literature. Jane Austen comes to mind. How can we not think of Mrs Bates and Miss Bates, and also Mr Woodhouse? And consider Jane's juvenilia. What about the mysterious stranger in 'Love and Freindship who finds he is the grandfather to a number of young people, and finding too he doesn't like them, he simply dispenses 50-pound notes and disappears' (Penguin Classics, 2015). Would the grandchildren have cared for him in later years? And Dickens causes Scrooge to care for Tiny Tim in *A Christmas Carol*. Maybe Tiny Tim will care for Scrooge when they are both older.

There's more to the literary influence, too, in Conduct manuals. These tell young women how to behave under all circumstances. Though I have yet to find one which fits care of elderly parents or other relatives into their chapters, I have found a number of manuals giving advice on caring for family, and presumably this could extend to the previous generation. For example, William Kenrick, with a new edition in 1753 of the work of Lady Mary Cressy in 1695, in *The Whole Duty of Woman* observes that 'Thy kingdom is thine own house, and thy government, the care of thy family.' P.(p'22) Presumably this would also include elderly.

And other records that tell a lot are those of the Poor Law documents. They ranged from the children's duty to visit, honour, and sometimes even financially assist (though not necessarily house) their mothers and fathers. Moreover, this duty was established by law: even if the law was seldom applied, the Poor Laws stipulated that children should support their aged parents.

Not only children, though, would be responsible for care. Although spouses and children occupied the most important positions as assistants to the aged, more distant kin such as siblings, grandchildren, cousins, nieces, and nephews, could play the important role of caregiver in the lives of their elderly relatives. Such data comes from both the diaries and wills that survive from the period. And this seems to be a stable pattern throughout the eighteenth century. From my reading of the numerous researchers listed above, it seems that there is no evidence of any change to family responsibility during this time. The elderly situations range from independent living to co-residence with families, either sharing the families' homes, or the families sharing the home of the elderly.

And in the family homes, the elderly can therefore still play their roles within the family setting, assisting in various ways, two of which are minding children, and financial help. Dependency is not something to be thought of at this juncture as both Thane and Ottaway say in their numerous publications.

Evidence from the household listings of the period shows considerable detail. And again I'm indebted to Susannah Ottaway (ibid.) for her detailed tables on 'Presence of children in households of individuals 6 and over' (p. 151) and 'Co-residents of individuals aged 60 plus, (aggregated by period and economic type, (p. 158). This latter includes grandchildren and 'Other non-nuclear kin:, lodgers and servants.'

These tables, among other relevant data, indicate the presence of available support within the household should the older person happen to need it, and it shows recognition of the mutual benefits that ensued when households were shared among generations. On the other hand, the study of household listings also shows that as individuals entered advanced old age, they became less likely to live with members of their families. Ottaway personalises these figures with interesting quotations (p. 162) from household listings from the various villages whose statistics she has already quoted. Details such as:

> Mary Chipp: a 66-year-old widow living in a household headed by her son. She is not in receipt of parish poor relief. Her son is a blacksmith, and he is married and they live with his 13-year-old illegitimate daughter. Mary knits, earning about 1s per week.

...and:

> Elizabeth Edmunds: a 66-year-old widow heading a household containing her son a 36-year-old carter, her daughter-in-law and her grandchildren aged 0-11, all of whom are listed as inmates rather than being in the "children" or "grandchildren" categories. Two of her grandchildren together

earn 3s 6d, while her son earns 7s. per week. None of them is listed as receiving parish poor relief.

And one more:

Reb Edmunds: a 54-year-old pauper widow who knits and heads a household with her son and daughter, aged 10 and 13, her grandson, aged 1/2 year, her daughter-in-law aged 27. All together the family earns about 6s. a week, and only Reb. is listed as receiving parish pay.

Although such sharing and reciprocity tends to be for those better off and higher in the social scale, as Ottaway says (Decline of Life, 2004), the above listings look to be towards the less well-off individuals. For the poorer and those even lower down the social scale it is more likely to see older individuals living in isolation from their close kin. So that where individuals were least able to support themselves, among the lower social strata, it was more likely that the older people were living in isolation despite the widely held belief that families should assist their elderly members. Nonetheless, there are details of isolated individuals becoming reliant upon their extended families (p. 166).

Kin was extremely important—a feature to note, which makes movements within the country and to other countries well worth considering in terms of care for family elderly.

For a close look at care I suggest we start at the bedside, where we see women involved in a wide range of caring and healing activities, many of these latter they preserved in one form of writing or another. Healing and remedies are a specialised form of care, but many caregivers would use home remedies, making them up themselves or getting from a neighbour who might be a healer in the community. Such care at home was helped by these home remedies. A note to look at Gerard's Herbal gives some idea of the number and sophistication of some of these herbal remedies.

Constant attention brings with it reactions by the caregivers, and depending on the number of caregivers, there could be both psychological and physical reactions, anger, miseries, exhaustion—to take some ideas from our own times.

So as well as the tasks of caregiving, we also need to know how various kin members dealt with their role as caregivers. In Chapter 4 of *Decline of Life*, Susannah Ottaway provides intriguing glimpses of emotions in kin relationships taken from the depth of her work with the diaries. Emotions such as 'attended to' by a father, mother described as 'the greatest temporal blessing; and on death of a father a great deal of affliction' noted.

Not everything was positive, though. We have a tale of a mother removing herself from visits to her son because she was offended. And there are other negativities in the descriptions of relationships, despite the moral obligations entailed on families to care. In-law relationships could be difficult. A mother-in-law, 'had a great volubility of tongue for invective, and especially if I am the subject.' And there are other such unpleasant comments from different families. Further unpleasantness reported is the disagreement between a widow and her newly widowed daughter-in-law over the division of the estate of the sun/husband' (Ottaway, ibid. p. 143).

Nor, of course, was it only the inter-relationship between two generations. Ottaway comments on grandchildren too, and on the wider network of kin. Unmarried sisters and brothers could be very useful to other members of their families.

As indeed could lodgers, for example, taken in to earn more money, or a wish for company, or even to maintain some independence from family members and from parish officers.

And I must say that there is much more. The above details have been quoted from Susannah Ottaway whose remarkable use of the diaries has painted such a clear picture of kin and care, as well as care and non-kin.

Care Itself

What I want it to look at now are the actual, factual situations as far as possible. Mary Fissell (2008) states:

> If we want to understand both women's involvement with healing, and how healing was on occasion gendered, we must focus on care. The very long periods of illness....entailed massive amounts of care, work that was often too ordinary or too unremarkable to be recorded in writing.

Various writers such as Susannah Ottaway, Mary Fissell, Montserrt Cabre, Monica Green, and Sandra Cavallo look at bodywork, or 'techniques of the body', or 'artisans of the body' and indicate that bodywork is most likely to be undertaken by women as already noted. So we can make a nod in the direction of women's role, women's work as Lesley Diack says in her doctoral dissertation and Barbara Caine comments (1997).

The problem can be in separating 'care' from nursing and healing. As Mary Fissell (2008) says in her Introduction, this was work that was often too ordinary or too unremarkable to be recorded in writing, but was usually performed by women: wives, mothers, daughters, domestic servants, and slaves. And, though not care itself, she talks too of 'searchers' who were 'elderly poor women hired by London's parishes to inspect the bodies of the sick and dead for signs of the dreaded plague' (p. 11). Not care itself, indeed no! But perhaps indicative of thought and care being taken on behalf of others.

Fissell also continues on the theme of bodywork and includes 'barbers and wigmakers' who, she says, 'existed at the boundaries of medicine, yet firmly within the category of bodywork' (p. 11) but that is another story, perhaps more in the medical category than that of caregiving. What Fissell offers is of considerable value, especially when she declares that

> If we want to understand both women's involvement with healing, and how healing was on occasion gendered, we must focus on care. The very long periods of illness....entailed massive amounts of care, work that was often too ordinary or too unremarkable to be recorded in writing, but was usually performed by women: wives, mothers, daughters, domestic servants, and slaves. The endless series of expulsive medicines, be they purges, vomits, or sweats, meant substantial quantities of nursing care and laundry. (p. 12)

In fact, though women were not allowed as physicians, many women were responsible for the health of their household, diagnosing, prescribing and preparing medicines at home. And Fissell is doing the job for us here. To underline the actions of care, she brings in the language used when caregivers were hired from parish women: this comes from records of the Old Poor Law, where the parish paid women and activities to 'do for', or 'help' or 'attend'.

These actions 'do for', 'help', 'attend' are remarkably general job descriptions for something so detailed as care.

Our view becomes clearer with more detail: bodywork and remedies; healing and care. Now we need to add that of 'place'.

Place—Home and Community—and Movement

Although community care was certainly present in previous eras, its visibility in the eighteenth century shows considerable personal detail as well as the general social concerns for the elderly. And though I want to highlight informal care at home, it's worth expanding our knowledge with some information on the growth of small institutions. Legislation and charity obligations recognised the needs of many more isolated elderly including those whose families were unable to care for them. The sources here are the statutes of the Poor Law, both old and new and the considerable pamphlet literature on poverty.

Through the functioning of these Poor Laws, and to a lesser extent, through charities, each parish in England recognized its need to shoulder the burden of its necessitous old inhabitants. This society's unshaken belief in the obligations of the 'collectivity' to its aged and infirm is reflected in the pamphlet literature surrounding the issues of poverty and the Poor Laws. The existence of the Old Poor Law meant that this sense of moral obligation was reinforced by widely used statutes of the realm. The evidence relevant to this issue reveals the striking continuity over the eighteenth century regarding expectations of community assistance for the elderly who were considered to be a particularly deserving category of the poor throughout this period. Ottaway (ibid) and Samantha Williams (1998) talk much of Poor Law help, and parish records show how the parishes took responsibility for the elderly poor, and assisted them to enter the local parish workhouse or almshouse, where they could take in a little work, and so build up some money for themselves. If that were not possible, then the poor or sick and disabled would live in a strictly regulated environment, where they were deprived of the personal freedom and choices which might have been previously available to them. The average age at entry into the workhouse was 70.1 years of age for elderly men, and 64.0 for aged women, and women often stayed in the workhouse for longer periods of time.

Living in institutions was not always easy. And it happened even to those with kin in the neighbourhood. No matter whether kin wanted to care or not, there were poverty and space issues and often their own suffering to prevent them from caring for their elder kin.

Who were these old people, forced to spend their final days in the parish workhouse? We would expect that these individuals would be the friendless and those without family in the parish but, as Ottaway shows in detail, many of the elderly had families living nearby, kin who could and might have cared for them but were unable to do so. With their children generally too poor to help them, these individuals were put into the workhouse regardless of the proximity of family members. In such cases, the importance of community over familial assistance is most obvious. And I am indebted again to Susannah Ottaway (ibid) for the following informative detail.

> Twenty-four of the thirty in Terling (80 percent) could be linked with certainty to a family reconstitution form (FRF), a form detailing the address, living situation and kin of the impoverished older person. And an additional two individuals had probable links to the FRFs,which means that they or their families were among the more settled poor whose life-cycle events were recorded in the parish registers. Of the entire group of individuals who received poor relief from 1771 to 1801, only 53 percent could be definitely linked to an FRF. Moreover, twenty-five of the individuals who eventually entered the workhouse in their old age had baptized children within the parish, so they were long-term residents. At least eleven, three women and eight men, definitely had children living in the parish of Terling during the years when they lived inside the workhouse. Others also certainly had children residing nearby, offspring who neither married nor died within the parish in the years of their parents' old age, and so left. (p. 254)

And we have from Mary Fissell's researches (1989) on the Bristol Infirmary that its clients often used the hospital to substitute for family structures. Old people with family connections were much more likely to remain outpatients than were their counterparts without local kin.' (p. 49). She also noted suggestive evidence on the Bristol Corporation for the Poor (essentially a workhouse) which also housed mostly elderly people who lacked nearby family. On the other hand, Alannah Tomkins found that of sixteen paupers who used the Shropshire Infirmary in the 1750s, seven had close relatives in Shrewsbury, two had no relatives, and seven were of unknown family situation..

I suggest that we can further embed care within the larger framework of healing and what various authors such as Kathy Brown. quoted in Fissell's work (ibid.) has called 'bodywork',which overlaps with Montserrat Cabré's and Monica Green's term, 'techniques of the body', and with Sandra Cavallo's suggestions about artisans of the body. Using bodywork as a basis, we still need to work out the details. Who does the actual washing, cleaning, help with pessaries and cups, help perhaps with prostheses, help with mobility? And how do caregivers cope with confusion, memory losses, cognitive impairments?

And although healing has not been in a definition of care, we might consider it as part of care of the household since many women grew and prepared herbal remedies, for use at home or for assisting others. Something to note, perhaps, in terms of healing and near-medical or medical practice.

References

Austen, Jane. originally pub. 1790. *Love and Freindship*. Penguin Classics, 2015.

Brown, Kathy. 2008. *Introduction: Women, Health and Healing in Early Modern Europe (Spring 2008)*, ed. Fissell, Mary, Vol. 82, no. 1, 1–17. Bulletin of the History of Medicine.

Cabre, Montserrat. 2000. From a Master to a Laywoman: A Feminine Manual of Self-Help (n. 13). *Dynamis: ActaHispanica adMedicinae Scieniiarumque Hisioriam lllustrandam* 20: 371–393.

Cavallo, Sandra. 2007. *Artisans of the Body in Early Modern Italy: Identities, Families and Masculinities*. Manchester: Manchester University Press.

Diack, Lesley. 1997. *English Feminism 1780–1980*, ed. Barbara Caine. OUP, Oxford.

Diack, Lesley. 1999. PhD dissertation, Women, Health and Charity: Women in the Poor Relief Systems in Eighteenth-Century Scotland and France (Aberdeen 1999).

Fissell, Mary. 1989. The 'Sick and Drooping Poor' in Eighteenth-Century Bristol and Its Region. *Social History of Medicine 2*(1) (April): 35–58.

Fissell, Mary. 2008. Introduction: Women, Health and Healing in Early Modern Europe (Spring 2008). *Bulletin of the History of Medicine 82* (1): 1–17.

Gleeson, Brendan. 1999. *Geographies of Disability*. Routledge.

Green, Monica. 2013. Caring for Gendered Bodies. In *Oxford Handbook of Medieval Women and Gender*, ed. Judith Bennett and Ruth mazo Karras, 345–361. Oxford : Oxford University Press.

Green, Monica. 2005. Bodies, Gender, Health, Disease: Recent Work on Medieval Women's Medicine in Studies in Medieval and Renaissance. *History* 2: 1–46.

History of Scotland. https://www.historic-uk.com/HistoryUK/HistoryofScotland/The-Highland-Clearances/ 1750.

Kuskey, Jessica. 2016. *The Working Body: Reforming the Factory Body*, Vol. 42, No. 1 Spring. Victorian Review, John Hopkins University Press.

Ljuslinder, Karin, et al. 2020. Cripping Time: Undertanding the Life Course through the Lens of Ableism. Umeå University, Faculty of Arts, Department of Culture and Media Studies. (DISLIFE) ORCID iD: 0000-0001-6671-4514.

Looser, Devoney. 2005. *A Companion to the Eighteenth-Century English Novel and Culture*, ed. Paula Backscheider and Catherine Ingrassia, 304. Australia: John Wiley & Sons.

Oliver, Michael, and Colin Barnes. 2012. *The New Politics of Disablement: 2nd Edition*, 52–73. Palgrave Macmillan.

Ottaway, Susannah. 2004. *The Decline of Life*. Cambridge UK: Cambridge University Press.

Ottaway, Susannah, and Samantha Williams. 1998. Reconstructing the Life-Cycle Experience of Poverty in the Time of the Old Poor Law. *Journal of the British Records Association 23*(98) (Kan. 1998).

Quadagno, Jill S. 1982. *Ageing in Early Industrial Society> Work, Family, and Social Policy in Nineteenth-Century England*, 20. Academic Press.

Sbaraini, E. 2021. *The Ageing Body, Memory-Loss and Suicide in Georgian England*. Social History of Medicine.

Smollett, Tobias. The Expedition of Humphry Clinker (1771, republished 2009). Oxford World Classics.

Tomkins, Alannah. 1999. Paupers and the Infirmary in Mid-Eighteenth-Century Shrewsbury. *Journal of Medical History 43*(2): 208–227.

Thane, Pat. 2002. *Old Age in English History: Past Experiences, Present Issues*. Oxford University Press.

Thane, Pat, and Lynn Botelho. 2005. *The Long History of Old Age*. Thames and Hudson Ltd.

Wrigley, E. 1966. *An Introduction to English Historical Demography from the Sixteenth to the Nineteenth Century*, editor. London : Weidenfeld & Nicolson.

CHAPTER 9

America—Eighteenth and Nineteenth Centuries

Introduction

And now time travel takes us to Nineteenth-century America for a number of reasons. As well as the major Indigenous tribes in North America, we have settlers from Europe—British, French, Spanish, and Dutch from the fifteenth century onwards. And as well as these European settlements, we also have that of enforced movement and settling of slaves. So nineteenth-century America is a multi-cultural country.

And there is much to be learned. My main reason for this selection and inclusion into the Westernised European information is not only the origin and the movement of the settlers but also there are informative and accessible sources that can provide some personal information which I want. Diaries and letters will provide us with the feelings of providing care and a look-see into inter-relationships arising from situations. And the care of slaves for themselves is of major interest—not only were slaves the subject of enforced movement but they are also forced into a way of life which, in care terms anyway, contrasted with their home lives as they themselves grow older.

And so, as much a product of movement as of increasing literacy in the population, we have considerable personal information from colonial America. We now have stories of caregiving revealing not only the mundanities of care but also the emotions, both positive and negative,

B. Hale, *Historical Reflections on Care in the Western World*,
https://doi.org/10.1007/978-3-031-87128-3_9

the personal strengths of the caregiver, and the need for help, as well as reaching out for help.

So we have here a valuable individual view of giving care, and not just to the care needs at home but also reaching out to the care in the community. This is better documented than in previous chapters and is a highly significant part of caregiving. It clearly demonstrates the skills and knowledge of the women required as caregivers, as well as their compassion and willingness to reach out and, perhaps later, expecting to receive some reciprocal activity.

I highlight as far as possible as a separate entity the slave population, how their elderly were treated, and cared for.

Ageing at This Time

How the general population regarded older people in early America is as varied as in previous times and countries. And we need to remember the incredible changes such as 'the political upheavals experienced by settlements north of Boston, as well as religious conflict and four devastating wars', as Laurel Thatcher Ulrich notes in *Good Wives* (p. 3).

According to David Hacket Fisher (1978), there were two sets of perceptions of the elderly: the first was a seventeenth- and eighteenth-century 'exalted' view of the elderly. Then from about 1780 onwards, this view deteriorated into the perception of a failing social status with new laws forcing retirement age and, among other things, (p. 88) there was considerable abuse in the language, instead of respect as had formerly been the case. And he pointed out that there was considerable gerontophobia in literature.

Clearly, not every older person was regarded with respect and how this affected the situation of care depends both on systematic considerations and undoubtedly on individual situations. Close reading of care arrangements made by elderly and ageing parents who have sons to inherit, suggest that older people wanted to ensure good care. Does such detail infer such insecurity and fears so much that care had to be spelt out? Remembering previous societies, and ancient Greece, in particular, older people might well feel insecure about children caring for them. But it's particularly interesting to note the emphasis on detail in the contractual care arrangements made by elderly and ageing parents with inheritor sons. Some things don't change: recollections of ancient societies remind us, particularly from Greek information, of possessions and property passing to family members and remaining in the family.

Reading such texts for colonial America suggests that reciprocity is one method by which the older people wanted to ensure their care.

Ulrich (ibid.) writing on 'ordinary women' and on the 'pots and pans history' describes the value of reciprocity but also finds that both elderly and younger women were sometimes the victims of family violence.

We need to know who were the overseers of such care, to ensure that care was carried out, and perhaps to stop violence.

Issues of Ageing

The issues of ageing and details of health and illness are similar to those we have already considered in previous chapters. Although human needs are known to change with varying contexts, certain issues do not change, and were brought with the settlers to America. For example, arthritis and heart problems are universal, and we could include dementia, though not yet known by that name, along with wounds and their results in the veterans of warfare. An example of these latter is written in the 1873, Consolidation Act which extended compensation to veterans for 'service-related conditions or diseases that later caused disabilities such as noise induced hearing loss, heart disease, and chronic bronchitis arising from pneumonia. Veterans, though certainly not confined to colonial America, were well treated cared for in terms of pensions. Nevertheless, such diseases and conditions were prevalent in other older people as well.

There were other chronic and incurable problems, and there might have been differences for the caregivers between the two. The diaries and letters we can read are drawn from the wealthier and more literate classes, but research shows a number of impoverished elderly and their families, and the comments are often on a hierarchy of merits, from the 'worthy' to the 'unworthy' who are so as a result of immorality, alcohol abuse, and laziness. Or so it was claimed at that time. Detail (p60)from Rochefort and Cobb in 1992 provides a vivid context. Those without close kin who were considered 'worthy' and were unable to support themselves through no fault of their own, due maybe to sickness, disability, or simply 'old age', received assistance in the form of institutional care.

A brief consideration of formal care shows us Erin Blakemore (2018) that the moral viewpoint in the community was that fear of the poor-house was believed to be the key to maintaining the work ethic among labourers and the poor. Although few questioned that elderly paupers deserved public assistance, shame and fear stigmatized all those on relief, worthy or not. Dread of life in an institution seems to be almost universal, although the most dreaded was, of course, the poorhouse. And a lack of family members willing or able to care for an elderly relative could result in the elderly individual moving to the poorhouse.

A brief description of this institution makes it clear that kin where they exist are by far the best to give care. Designed to dissuade the undeserving poor' from seeking relief, poorhouses provided a meagre existence. Residents were known as 'inmates', and some work was expected of all but the most frail. How much care existed in the poorhouse for the elderly is debatable and fragmented. There were some alternatives to the almshouses or poorhouses. For example, urban Catholic churches and Jewish communities built homes for 'superannuated immigrant congregants'. But these were not universal go-to homes for chronically ill elderly.

For care, clearly, kin was by far the best.

Home Space

In a blog, 'Discovering lives', Paula Tarnapoll Whiteacre (2025) has provided some fascinating information about caregiving duties, referring to Julia Wilbur as a dutiful daughter. Julia's life was one of caregiving from age 19 when her mother died and she assumed the care of nine younger siblings. This care continued as these needed more and different help, on marriage, childbirth, and sickness. But Julia carried on with her own life as far as possible, though continuing to care, especially for her 'enfeebled' father. And as Whiteacre said, 'In the 1800s the home was the optimal center of care for the sick and elderly.'

Isolation is often a component of neglect, but unlike some elderly in mediaeval and Renaissance England, the elderly in this society were generally not left alone. Households seem to have been fluid in terms of personnnel, and despite the older person's anxieties, it appears that the elderly were likely to be cared for, at least in the sense of being part of a group, and therefore not isolated. Children move out, boarders/lodgers move in, to be cared for if needed, and children might move back because of economic necessity. An elderly person living alone could move in as a boarder to alleviate the isolation and this leads us to consider this fluid household as a potential care situation. It seems that lodger/boarder type situations are common during this era as well as in previous times.

Older people in this situation were unlikely to be pushed into isolation and segregation. And such flexible households certainly suggest companionship at least. One question to be asked is whether these elderly were active enough to take on a role within the household or whether they were passive and required care.

Household data from various studies suggest considerable interdependence among family members, whether voluntary or forced, and there are statistics in support of this contention. In urban areas, 64% of older men lived with adult offspring, and over 90% of these were heads of household, while more than 70% of older women living with adult offspring were either heads or spouses of heads, and the suggestion is that in the cities older people retained at least titular control of their families. The results of numerous historical investigations suggest a variety of intergenerational relationships and this should have its effect on caregiving.

Control could be as simple as financial, and as complex as childcare if the mother had to work, or in supervising/organising household arrangements.

And further information tells us that the number of older people co-residing with non-kin is about one-third of the aged population, living as friends or lodgers. Whether these figures from Essex County are similar to other areas of the country is something to be considered, but it does give an insight into living arrangements and possible care arrangements.

Kinresidences were about 20–30 per cent older men and 30–40 per cent older women and about less than half the men and one-third of the women resided in nuclear family homes.[1] What this can mean for care needs and caregiving is that there is an emerging picture of households with people around to help, and presumably greater care was forthcoming when needed. Who cared for whom has not been clarified but it is possible that lodgers were taken in order to care for the landlady/lord, and that friends cared for each other.

Clearly care doesn't just happen; it appears to be the result of conscious planning and forethought.

Similarly, the timing of later life transitions affected more than one generation. For example, the death of 'old, old' parents enabled caretaking children who were themselves old to begin providing for their own old age, as well as for adult children or grandchildren (Hogan quoted in Hareven, 1994).

In concluding this section we see the expectations of adult children were to be the main caregivers for their ageing parents, and the length of time was expected as a short one, given the high mortality rate. Families were committed to kin care, and mutual assistance was not strictly calculative with such assistance being reciprocal with children and across generations. It seems in general that caring individuals did so from duty and familial obligation, rather than expecting immediate gain. There were, of course, protests and competition and conflict among siblings as to who should carry the main responsibility of support, as we will see from the personal information quoted later in the chapter.

Competition and conflict are understandable since the duties of care could be considerable, and the length of time incalculable, though generally felt to be shorter rather than longer, given the high mortality rates of the elderly, so caregiving was not necessarily a lengthy period of time.

But what is it carers actually did? What did it feel like to 'give care', to be a caregiver? And what was the social position of anyone who was a caregiver? Presumably, there were servants or slaves assisting to, for example, empty commodes, bring wash water, ensure clean sheets and clothing. But also, women of 'diverse social strata'[2] 'administered medications, applied poultices, watched for dangerous symptoms, changed dressings, and cleaned up vomit, excrement, and pus.' (Abel, 2000, p. 37).

Formal Care?

The institutions of almshouses, workhouses, and rural 'poor farms' were intended to take in the poor and helpless as I mentioned earlier in the chapter. These had existed since colonial times as both a refuge for the helpless and a deterrent to the able-bodied. Assistance to poor people was based on the assumption that the recipient must be truly incapacitated for work and the dying poor were shunted to institutions, which certainly increased their misery and likely hastened their deaths.

Community leaders took responsibility here by paying for housing for the homeless. If unable to live on their own, then they were housed in what was described as a 'foster care setting'. If they were able to live on their own, the counties provided them with funds to get shelter, feed and clothe themselves.

This was a public event. Many recipients of county assistance had to wear a red or blue letter "P" on their chest which stood for poverty, alerting all to their misfortune.

People had to be almost desperate before seeking and gaining entry to any of these institutions. Details from researchers such as Michael Katz (1996) describe poorhouses as dreaded, with residents known as 'inmates' and expected to work and contribute to the living in the poorhouse.

Legalities

Space was only one element. There was also finance to be considered. One example comes from Laurel Thatcher Ullrich (ibid.) where widowed Judith Coffin received a comfortable maintenance, rather than traditional 'thirds'. Son Nathaniel, the youngest, was 'to take spesshall care' of his mother to 'provid for har in all Respectes'. The other sons were to help, paying their brother a fixed sum annually for their mother's support.

And as well as the financial aspect, there were legalities involved, as there had been in the past. Ageing parents had to enter into contracts with their inheriting sons in order to secure support in old age in exchange for land. The emphasis in such arrangements on specific details suggests the potential tensions and insecurities that parents anticipated concerning their care after they became too frail to support themselves, says John Demos. Hareven (1978) supports these data saying that historians have uncovered conscious strategies underlying inheritance contracts in rural society, in which sons agree to support ageing parents in exchange for inheriting property.

Personal

However many examples we can find to give us some inklings about ensuring care and giving care, the best way of finding out is to ask the caregivers. When this is impossible, look up diaries and letters. Also careful reading of court texts will provide enough material to infer the situation of the caregiver. We are fortunate to have some exceptional material for nineteenth-century America.

To make a start with the personal here, I want to describe the situation of Emily Gillespie. And this material has been quoted from Emily Abel's work, *Hearts of Wisdom* (2000), from the first part of this book.

J'ames Gillespie and Emily were married in 1863. They were farmers in 19th century Iowa, and she had a busy working life. They had two children, Sarah and Henry.'

James had mental health problems. He suffered from major depressions and 'uncontrollable rages' and Emily was terrified of him, as well as angry at his mistreatment and brutality when he was physically well, and sadness when he was sick, with his mental illness. Her relationship with her husband fluctuated from love and sadness when he was well to fear and anger. As for caring, what she did was put up with him in his mental disorders, and when physically ill, she did the hands-on caring, rubbing his 'stummick with linament'.

Not only does she build caring into her numerous tasks at home, but also her diary shows some movement within the community and slightly further afield, when she visits her sister to help on her farm, and her son when he has an accident. But caregiving takes place also in the community by herself or in company with her friends.] For example, she writes, 'Mrs Houghton and I sat up all last night with old Mrs Stephens, 74, she died ten minutes past nine this morning. We lay her out in black dress. I came home this morning.' And this was only one of many such occasions. A vivid description from Emily, summoned to help her wounded uncle, was 'about 3 inches flesh, bones, arteries, cords and all had to be removed' from her uncle's arm. She continued to help him. And there are many other stories of Emily's outreach.

And still in this first part of Abel's work, when Emily herself was sick:

> [...] was real sick all night (last night) did not sleep a minute...about daylight James sent for some help to take care of me. Pa went, got Mrs Lewis, Mrs Coats, Mrs Parliman and Margaret. Ma (James' mother) was here. The occasion was the birth of baby Henry, and Mrs Lewis was the Dr (paid her $2.00) she is a real good woman.

So Emily was a caregiver and care receiver within her farming community and, later, her daughter Sarah followed her example. At the same time, it is clear that while Emily offered care, others helped her in her need.

Also to be considered here is dealing with spacious environment of the farms and their distance from each other. Crossing such space took time, and we have to remember that transport then was horseback, or horse and carriage. Slow, much slower obviously than a car. Not only could lack of transport delay the doctor's arrival but would also prevent easy ongoing care and supervision by the medic concerned. And this, of course meant that the caregiver had to manage by herself, or with the help of neighbours. And neighbours had to take time out of their own daily routines to give such help.

Not only do we have detail from the Gillespies, but we also have *The Diary of Elizabeth Drinker*, subject of a thesis by Catherine Teets-Parzynski from LeHigh University who also is the subject of a book edited by Elaine Forman Crane (2010).

Gleanings? Soundings?

What can we take from these descriptions for the carer role?

We can underline the fact of carer knowledge and expertise, due not only to the expense of medical health care, but also to the spatiality of the area, where regular frequent medical visits and call-outs were difficult. The women learned from each other, and were as expert in caring for chronic illness and disability as any trained professional.

So, spatially we have care at home and care in the community. This brings us to an interchange of knowledge, expertise, goodwill, and giving and accepting help—and so we also have the notion of reciprocity. Reciprocity is prominent and neighbourly help was important since, without the modern inventions of telephones and cars and now the internet, requesting the attendance of physicians involved considerable time and effort. And such physicians were expensive. Hence to be able to call on your neighbours for ideas, information, knowledge, practical help, and support was of great importance.

Time also enters into our carerscape, less in terms of measuring against immediate productivity, but in terms of the caregiver's own life course. Sarah Gillespie is the prime example here, of giving up teaching to care for her mother. Such sacrifices may be detrimental both to the caregiver's own finances and to her career. Julia Wilbur, reported in Paula Tarnapo Whitacre's blog, however, did not give up her life to care—an interesting contrast to many carers.

We therefore have to introduce economics into caregiving: the cost to the caregiver might be considerable. What might be the cost to the work-force itself? Further insights into the economies in caregiving come from Tamara Hareven's (ibid.) (2013). research into 'Essex County in 1873–1880' where she found that there was considerable economic pressure. She suggests that 'people tightened intergenerational bonds, and situations of reciprocal assistance rather than dependency emerged.' And the practicalities of ageing and sharing your house with your adult children is using the house as a commodity, in exchange for assistance and possibly care.

And there is some financial information from the Gillespie diaries, where the notion of independence or rather, lack of independence, was introduced. There seems to have been no other recourse for Emily Gillespie but to care for her husband in his bad times (though the literature on the diaries query some of the statements, I intend to take the diary as it is written and reported by Emily Abel in her first chapter.)

Dependency emerges from one of Abel's observations from Emily's comments was that she had to continue with farming for their income, and possibly felt herself to be reasonably autonomous, if that was an interpretation to be considered at that time. But she was not independent, and the question arises as to what independence or dependence might mean. Emily was dependent on her husband for income, on her daughter for eventual care, on her neighbours to help her or she to help them, which provided her with some camaraderie and friendship.

And this of course brings us to another question: how did these aspects affect their relationships with the health professionals.

Sarah Gillespie—Her Turn

But return to the diaries and read what daughter Sarah did for her mother Emily when Emily appeared 'sickly' and her hands were 'numb' said Sarah. Emily herself thought that the relationship stresses had created her health problems. (And when Emily was sick, Sarah was torn between her pleasure in her own growing independence and teaching work, and caring for her mother Such care required 'rubbing and hot flannels, hot teas' and round the clock care, caring for her mother between two and six times each night. Emily Abel writes vividly of Sarah and her duties in Chapter One.

Sarah's primary duty was a daughter and a woman and therefore was the principal person to provide this care, and it was a labour of love, because she loved her mother. But she also longed to be back teaching at school.

And Sarah was the primary caregiver, since her father refused to help at all. Their relationship deteriorated, as we can see from her written comments which talk of her feelings about her father's unwillingness to help. When Sarah asked James to help, James responded by telling her not to bother him and her diary comments were that 'I thot I needed rest if any one'.

Sarah's relationship with her father, as well as Emily's with James, opens up an exploration of relationships for caregivers. Initially, caregiving is a dyad; gradually others are brought into this, expanding the relational environment, if you like, to neighbours and to professional helpers, as we have already mentioned.

But what about relationships with other kin? Could they assist? Or did they need themselves?

For the Gillespies, these relationships were initially positive but deteriorated later when Harriet's husband failed to provide for his family. Emily travelled to help them when needed, in care terms. Emily was angry with her sister for demanding so much from her when she (sister) was sick or in childbirth. She was also angry with her father whom she suspected of taking too much from her when he came to live with her, to be cared for when needed, and of colluding with her sister. The relationships among the three make interesting reading.

Other stories of caregiving show the detail of extended kin care, and the spirit of caregiving in the community, with obligations and reciprocity foremost, and underlying these is the extent of the knowledge which caregivers have. Of interest here perhaps is the observation by Daniel Blackie (2014) that family as we know it today was, in the American nineteenth century, a household of co-residents, the composition of the household not necessarily being of kin.

If we go further back into history, soldiers wounded in the Civil War counted on families both to journey to them and rescue them and also to care for them. There is a story about a 73 year old veteran, James Trowbridge, who was 'laid up' for years because of his war wounds, and during this time he was cared for by his much younger wife whose health was 'ruined' by caring for him, as he acknowledged.

Another story, not war-related this time is of a niece caring for two aunts. The second is a neighbourhood situation. The space of caring is now beyond the home and household.

Again from Emily Abel (ibid) we have the information that in 1867, Laura Stebbens was unable to join a friend in reform work, because she was caring for her nearly eighty year old aunt who was frail and feeble—and both of her aunts are helpless.... Laura goes on to say that 'if they suffered from illness or accident, I should reflect upon myself exceedingly.'

And quotes from Nannie Stillwell Jackson from her published diary of life in the rural south 1890 and 1891 shows details of neighbourhood obligations. Nannie exchanged goods and services with at least 20 other women, both white and African American. She was active in care for sick and dying people, and often 'set a while' with two boys of a friend, both of whom were sick. When 'Mrs Dyer' was afflicted with boils, Nannie visited her. Nannie and Fannie spent time with Mrs Caulk when her baby was ill. When Mrs Archdale (mother of the boys) was sick, Nannie gave her 'a dose of oil and turpentine and some gum camphor'. And when she became worse, Nannie visited her '5 or 6 times' and she and Fannie spent the night with her. When she died, Nannie and several neighbours 'dressed her and laid her out'.

Sarah, again from Abel, also helped care for her brother Henry when, as the result of an accident, he was bedridden and 'fanned and rubbed every second by myself and Ma….we had to work so hard just to keep him alive.' Sarah's diaries are preserved in the Iowa State Historical collection, and well worth keeping, being so informative.

But not all caring was seven days a week, 24 hours a day, hands-on bodily care. Some of it was intermittent, some temporary, and some caregiving ended with the death of the cared-for person.

So, although this is not care for the chronic illness/long-term ageing situation, we have a more vivid description of hands-on care at home than we have had previously. Furthermore, these women spread their knowledge and skills into outreach within their local communities, sitting up with ill and dying patients, helping with childbirth and assisting in various ways with the nursing, hands-on caring.

Since the role is obviously initially a kinship role, these women could perhaps be described as fictive kin. And maybe because of the nature of migration, the creation of 'fictive kin' became customary where women participated in 'mutual aid', no doubt to be sociable and friendly, and also perhaps, as Abel comments (p. 38), as a form of insurance. This sounds remarkably familiar to a migrant from the UK in late twentieth-century New Zealand. Mutual aid in terms of babysitting, transport, help of various sorts, was very much in the role of migrant stay-at-home wives. You gave, and in turn, you received.

Since migration often meant separation, as well as distance, what happens in situations where more care help is needed? Care in and by the community is important, as we noted above. We have another two examples to set beside what the Gillespie women achieved.

The first is a niece caring for two aunts. The second is a neighbourhood situation. Space of caring is now beyond the immediate home and household.

The skills of these caregivers were invaluable and relationships among them would have been an interesting study with exchange of ideas and information, teaching each other different skills, perhaps. Whether such relationships were always positive is also a matter of interest.

However, there are also relationships with health professionals and alternative health professionals and because of the distance factor, no doubt such relationships were limited.

Occasionally they stopped by the house, left medicine, discussed the prognosis and offered advice. But such visits were rare.

It is a feature of caregiving that there are relationships with others involved with health care, informal or formal. And this can be seen in *The Diary of Elizabeth Drinker*, who gave freely and willingly to those who needed help. Two examples are:

When Susannah Swett was no longer able to live independently as a result of old age, Drinker took her in until suitable accommodations could be found. And when Hannah Shoemaker was suffering with breast cancer, it was Elizabeth who helped her through her mastectomy.

One of the most fascinating descriptions is of Elizabeth learning to create home remedies, by watching others work, getting advice and recipes from friends, and from reading. A healer and a carer.

Conclusion

What do we take from the information in this part of the chapter?

From the section on 'gleaning' I have listed items such as economics, reciprocal time, and relationships. Spatiality brings us a vocabulary of distance, having to drive to see and help family. Add to this vocabulary of distance, we have community and neighbourhood, reaching out to give and to receive help. Add too, the difficulties of getting professional medical care, because of such distances, which in itself has some influence on relationships with the knowledgeable, experienced and on-the-spot caregiver. Family care and the emotional elements are much more clearly spelt out.

And the visibility of caregiving, I suggest, is becoming greater, even though much of it was done unseen at home by home- or farm-based women. But many of the early American women were literate and professional women, having been trained to teach.

To give that up, or to incorporate caregiving and work makes the action of caring more visible.

At the same time, society was permitting, encouraging perhaps, the expression of emotions—maybe this is social movement, and maybe too it is the advent of literacy, coupled with the availability of writing materials.

Part 2—Slaves

And while we are in America, we should look at the situation of slaves, their ageing and care for themselves. Caregiving in slave conditions has to contend with similar factors but with a difference: home influence, distance, work environment under authority, and a belonging to the slave community.

The main focus on elder care in slavery times involves both black families and white 'owners', Our information here is from a repository of oral information taken from griots (or troubadour–historians rooted in West African culture). These West African historians or Indigenous oral historians were highly respected as repositories of cultural historical beliefs, legends, and facts. Griot information said that their families traditionally treat black older adults with great respect. To link this with the spirits, the ancestral worship of the West Africans, the group with whom we are dealing, contains a belief that older adults are closest to their ancestors. This belief helps contribute to respect for the living elderly. The line of kinship is a strong one, and the weight of knowledge and approval of the past is a powerful influence. This tradition extends from known customs of pre-slavery civilizations on the African continent through to modern customs among African American families and kinship groups in the United States. This custom is similar to that of the Chinese, who have traditionally venerated their aged, believing they were but one step removed from a spiritual union with their ancestors.[3=]

Using slaves was clearly an economic interest for the white slave owners, and we have to ask how did the African slaves maintain their respect for their elderly, under slave labour conditions. Were families kept together? Sometimes yes, often not. How did families manage to maintain care and respect for elderly according to their spiritual beliefs and traditions?

Was there care for ageing slaves, and those with disabilities? Did the slave owners care for their ageing slaves? The situation of elderly disabled slaves was especially tenuous, in particular the act of emancipating old slaves, which was seen as a means of escaping responsibility for them. The Whites of Maryland expressed outrage at the extent to which slaveholders were emancipating their old slaves in order to escape responsibility for them.

The economics of caregiving competed with the economic interests of the slave owners. An example from Baltimore, and true too of other southern cities, was the focus of freed country Blacks, who then became a public charge. The residents of the southern cities fought for tough laws to curb this practice. No less staunch a pro-slavery writer than Dr Josiah Mott of Mobile revealed the fragility of paternalistic concerns in his attack on the practice of insuring slaves.

> As long as the Negro is sound, and worth more than the amount insured, self-interest will prompt the owner to preserve the life of the slave; but, if the slave became unsound and there is little prospect of perfect recovery, the underwriters cannot expect fair play—the insurance money is worth more than a slave, and the latter is regarded rather in the light of a superannuated horse. (Genovese, 1974, p. 520)

This quotation was followed by the comment that some urban slaveholders solved the problem of old, disabled slaves by sending them out to peddle or beg to bring in some income as well as support themselves.

Insofar as white caretakers or owners were concerned, the antebellum (pre-Civil War) treatment of old, disabled Blacks ranged from full and kind concern to minimum attention to paternalism. In the negative extreme, there was indifference and sheer physical and mental abuse.

Manumission may or may not have been an exceptional way of treating older slaves. Whatever its frequency, it was certainly not the only response to the old and disabled. It was disturbing to find such details in archival research, although not surprising after reflection on the investment economy in slavery, where it was seen that slavers quite often sought to sell or trade their old disabled slaves and acquire younger 'stock' for fear of losing the investment they had made. One account reported that the appearance of 'old slaves' was sometimes 'doctored up', made to look younger than they actually were before they were sold. Youthful appearances would bring a better price.

Immigrants and Blacks had the fewest resources for old age. Statistics say that by 1850, 3.8% of Blacks were older than 60 years and 1.4% was older than 70 years. The vast majority were slaves, unable to hold property or generate savings. Elderly slaves were sometimes freed before they became a burden to the plantation, but they were denied food and shelter and were left to starve. Recall by one former slave, Moses Grandy, wrote

> When my mother became old, she was sent to live in a little lonely log-hut in the woods. Aged and worn out slaves, whether men or women, are commonly so treated. No care is taken of them, except, perhaps, that a little ground is cleared about the hut, on which the old slave, if able, may raise a little corn. As far as the owner is concerned, they live or die as it happens; it is just the same thing as turning out an old horse.... She was not treated worse than others: it is the general practice. (https://docsouth.unc.edu/fpn/grandy/grandy.html)

Although abandonment was discouraged in some regions, senescence did not reduce the owner's demand for labour, and few slaves were allowed to retire; some were given menial tasks, and others were sold. Auction and plantation records document that elderly slaves were sold as mere fractions of a 'full hand'.

But among slaves themselves, there was a culture of respect for older slaves, according to Frederick Douglass, lest they risk severe reprimand. 'A Young slave must approach the company of the older with hat in hand, and woe betide him, if he fails to acknowledge a favour of any sort, with the accustomed "tank'ee".'

The bonds and customs of deference among slaves, no doubt, functioned as sources of social and psychological support for old disabled slaves, facilitating their coping with the harsh and inhumane demands of the slavers' culture. Included among the means by which older slaves supported and cared for each other's health was folk medicine.

Support for older adults was also provided by younger able-bodied slaves who shared their 'wages' or whatever they gleaned from their labour with the older disabled who were less able to fend for themselves.

David Brion Davis, who has written considerably on slavery in America, emphasizes the support which older slaves gave to younger, whether kin or not, and presumably this would be reciprocated, when the older slaves were ill or disabled—should care of these be allowed by the slave masters.

Reading about care brings in family and close non-kin, or we might term it community. To compare slaves with white women it is obvious that although many white women were caregivers and had major issues with this, at least they could look after their own family members. Slave women always had to put their owners' demands first. Although slave families were highly vulnerable as an institution—liable to be broken up by various members being sold off to other white slave masters in different areas—there was still the semblance of older to younger care and interaction, telling of old stories, of tribal beliefs, one of which was care and respect for the older generation as David Brion Davis repeatedly emphasizes.

Caregiving was especially likely to solidify women's support networks. It was even more common for enslaved women than for white women to render care without male assistance. On the basis of a statistical analysis of slave households in twenty-six Louisiana parishes, as Ann Malone (2000) supports this with her comments on the matrifocal element in slavery, at some stages more so than contemporary white families.

Women shared healing knowledge as well as responsibilities and younger women learned from their elders. Harriet Collins remembered, 'All dese doctorin' things come clear from Africy, and dey allus worked for mammy and for me, too;.'

And many other former slaves credited their African-born grandmothers with transmitting healing lore. This information is spread widely in discussions of slaves and slavery, and Daniel Barber's thesis (2015) on African Medical Culture in slave times is a good place to start.

Then Malone goes on to discuss medical beliefs and rituals…and practitioners (often men) variously known as conjurers, root doctors and hoodoos used spiritual forces to harm as well as heal. Laurie A.Wilkie, (1995), comes information on conjurers root doctors, hoodoos. But religious beliefs also infused more routine forms of care from of care. As Sharla Fett (2002) write that caring was most often practised by women, as nurses, or herbalists and also general daily domestic care. And that these were part of African part of a continuum of African American healing resources which drew upon notions of spiritual power…These notions included the beliefs that illnesses stemmed from metaphysical as well as natural causes'.

> The dying person was surrounded by the community who offered comfort and support… Singing, praying and pious conversation filled the cabin

> nightly. In Herbert C. Covey (2007) Janey Landrum, a former slave in Texas recalled (p.34), 'The neighbours come in and help nurse when there was sickness in the family.' Crowded habitations facilitated the collective nature of caregiving.

Abel (2000, p. 37 ff) cites a 'web of mutual obligations bound enslaved people to grandparents, grandchildren, aunts, uncles, nieces, nephews and siblings, while "fictive kinship' linked unrelated individuals to each other, enhancing communal solidarity. Collective care for sick and disabled people may in turn, have reinforced the bonds of kinship and community that sustained whatever dignity and joy enslaved people achieved.'

Stories

To conclude this part of the chapter, I quote a slave story from Dea Boster

Dorothy's positioning as a response to disability increases in intensity when more disabled family members are added 'When the four of us kids got old enough to fend for ourselves, Dorothy was starting to think her usefulness with us had come to an end. But then the house filled up with Grandpa and Sister and she was needed even more' (p. 91).

And again taken from Dea Boster,

> This language of usefulness is rhetorically reminiscent of slavery discourses which Dea Boster identifies as focused on similar kinds of 'usefulness' and 'uselessness,' particularly regarding slaves' abilities and disabilities. Dorothy is 'useful' to the Karasiks in her ability to respond to disability and normalize family functioning. This assumes that Dorothy is completely devoted to the family, saddened by not being useful anymore, and thrilled when her services are needed unexpectedly for an elderly grandfather and intellectually disabled aunt. In this way, Dorothy is characterized as reminiscent of the loyal and obedient mammy figure, both as a response to or amelioration of disability, and as I explore, as potentially disabled body herself. (Shannon Walters, 2017)

And more stories:

> The young mistress came out to see how things were done on her plantation, and she soon gave a specimen of her character. Among those in waiting for their allowance was a very old slave, who had faithfully served the Flint family through three generations. When he hobbled up to get his

> bit of meat, the mistress said he was too old to have any allowance; that when niggers were too old to work, they ought to be fed on grass. Poor old man! He suffered much before he found rest in the grave.

And the next story:

> When my grandmother's illness became known, many ladies, who were her customers, called to bring her some little comforts, and to inquire whether she had everything she wanted. Aunt Nancy one night asked permission to watch with her sick mother, and Mrs Flint replied, "I don't see any need of your going. I can't spare you." But when she found other ladies in the neighbourhood were so attentive, not wishing to be outdone in Christian charity, she also sallied forth, in magnificent condescension, and stood by the bedside of her who had loved her in her infancy, and who had been repaid by such grievous wrongs. She had always slept on the floor in the entry, near Mrs Flint's chamber door, that she might be within call.

I have to ask: was this an aspect of care?

Conclusion

What do we take from the information in this chapter? Vocabulary of distance, for one thing, reporting on needs and care given. Family care and the emotional elements are much more clearly spelt out here in the diaries and letters. These colonists were literate and professional women, having been trained to teach. And they noted in their diaries and wrote letters.

The notion again, of community, neighbourhood, and reaching out to help, support, and care. And further, the notion of independence, linked with the concept of reciprocity.

At the same time, there was the growth and accessibility of magazines and many American magazines touched on such subjects of interest to women. There were in the first sixty years of the nineteenth century, more than twenty journals for women, general interest magazines and children's publications. Kinship responsibilities will have their place here.

And while I do not want to touch even the fringes of suffragism which is a huge topic—it is known that caregiving is emphasized as women's work. And alongside caregiving, keeping the rest of the household going, and maybe even the farm work/or self-employed businesses too.

At the same time society is permitting, encouraging perhaps, the expressions of emotions—maybe this is social movement, and maybe too it is the advent of literacy, coupled with the availability of writing materials.

Economics are important too both in the White and certainly the slave community. The financial value of caregiving to the individual, the lack of finance to the caregiver, and the value of the slaves deserve a book to themselves.

References

Abel, Emily K. 2000. *Hearts of Wisdom,: American Women Caring for Kin, 1850–1940*, Ch. 2, 37. Harvard University Press.

Abel, Emily K. 2022. For Stebbens, Laura *Looking to the Past, What the Nineteenth Century can tell us,* Elder Care in Crisis (2022). NYU Press.

Achenbaum, W. Andrew, and Christian L. Carr. 2014. *A Brief History of Aging Services in the United States*. American Society on Ageing Generations, Summer.

Barber, Daniel. 2015. African American Medical Culture in the Antebellum South as remembered in the WPA Narratives. Master's thesis, University of California.

Blackie, Daniel. 2014. Disability, Dependency and Family in the Early United States. In *Disability Histories, eds. Burch, Susan and Michael Rembis*. University of Illinois.

Blakemore, Erin. (2018). Poorhouses Were Designed to Punish People for Their Poverty. https://www.history.com/articles/in-the-19th-century-the-last-place-you-wanted-to-go-was-the-poorhouse

Boster, Dea. 2013. *African American Slavery and Disability: Bodies, Property and Power in the Antebellum South, 1800–1860*. New York: Routledge.

Collins, Harriet. Interview for Slavery in Texas, Slave Narratives, Vol. XVI, Part 1, https://slaveryintexas.org/items/show/127.

Covey, Herbert C. 2007. *African American Slave MedicineL Herbal and Non-herbal Treatment*. Lanham MD: Lexington Books.

Crane, Elaine Forman. 2010. *The Diary of Elizabeth Drinker*. Philadelphia: University of Pennsylvania Press.

Davis, David Brion. 1966. *The Problem of Slavery in Western Culture*. Ithaca, New York: Cornell University Press.

Demos, John. 1999. *Å Little Commonwealth: Life in Plymouth Colony*, 2nd ed. New York, NY: Oxford University Press.

Fett, Sharla. 2002. *Working Cures: Healing, Health and Power in Southern Slave Plantations*. Chapel Hill: University of North Carolina Press.

Fisher, James A. 1969. The Struggle for Negro Testimony in California 1851–1863. *Southern California Quarterly* 51: 313–324.

Fisher, David Hackett. 1978. *Growing Old in America, The Bland-Lee Lectures 1978*. USA: Oxford University Press.

Grandy, Moses. https://docsouth.unc.edu/fpn/grandy/grandy.html

Genovese, Eugene D. 1974. *Roll, Jordan, Roll: The World the Slaves Made,* Pantheon Books, U.S.

Hareven, Tamara K. 1978. *Transitions: Family and the Life Course in Historical Perspective*. New York, NY: Academic Press.

Hareven, Tamara K. 1979. From the Empty Nest to Family Dissolution: Life Course Transitions into Old Age. *Journal of Family History* 4 (1) (March): 69–83.

Hareven, Tamara K. 2013. ed. *Transitions: Family and Life Course in Historical Perspective,* Studies in Social Discontinuity, Academic Press

Jackson, Nannie Stillwell. 2025. *Vinegar Pie and Chicken Bread: A Woman's Diary of Life in the Rural South 1890–1891*, ed. Margaret Jones Bolsterli 1982. University of Arkansas Press.

Katz, Michael B. 1996. *In the Shadow Of the Poorhouse: A Social History Of Welfare In America* (https://www.hachettebookgroup.com/titles/michael-b-katz/in-the-shadow-of-the-poorhouse/9780465024520/?lens=basic-books). New York: Basic Books.

Kleinman, Arthur. 1989. *The Illness Narratives: Suffering, Healing and the Human Condition*. New York, NY: Basic Books.

Malone, Ann Patton. 2000. *Sweet Chariot: Slave Family and Household Structure in Nineteenth Century Louisiana*. Chapel Hill, NC: University of North Carolina Press.

Newman, S. L., and D. M. Turner. 2024. Disability, Gender and Old Age in the Industrial Revolution: Cultural Historical and Osteoarchaeological Perspectives. In *The Material Body: Embodiment, History and Archaeology in Industrialising England, 1700–1850*, ed. E. Craig-Atkins and K. Harvey, 205–235. (Social Archaeology and Material Worlds). Manchester University Press. https://doi.org/10.7765/9781526152794.00014

Rochefort, David, and Roger Cobb. 1992. Framing and Claiming the Homelessness Problem. *New England Journal of Public Policy* 8 (1).

Stone, Lawrence. 1977. 'Walking Over Grandma' review May 12th issue of the New York Review of Book.

Teets-Parzynski, Catherine, I Arose and Gave Him Mint Water, He Is Better Today: A Re-evaluation of Women's Roles in Domestic Medicine using the Diary of Elizabeth Sandwith Drinker, 1750–18390 (1995). Theses and Dissertations. Paper 34.

Ulrich, Laurel Thatcher. 1991. *Good Wives, Image and Reality in the Lives of Women in Northern New England, 1750*. NY: Knopf.

Walters, Shannon. 2017. Crip Mammy: Complicating Race, Gender and Care in *The Ride Together. Journal of Literary & Cultural Disability Studies 11*(4). https://doi.org/10.3828/jlcds.2017.36.

Whitacre, Paula Tarnapol. 2025. Discovering Lives, (blog).

Wilkie, Laurie A. 1995. Magic and Empowerment on the Plantation: an archaeological consideration of African—American World View—read online on Scribd.

CHAPTER 10

Sharing the Caregiving Experience: Soundings from the Media

The visibility of caregiving is now much stronger. But before I reinforce this visibility by moving on to contemporary factual information on caregiving; I want to undertake a little fictional journey, with maybe a sidestep into poetry and non-fiction. So many of these stories are immortal and, along with their main themes, they have established the existence and persistence of caregiving. Others make caregiving the main theme of the story.

And what emerges from past to present is the similarity in caregiving. I've made a list, with a few comments only, from only a few of the great writers and movie makers, including Shakespeare, Austen, Dickens, and others. Nothing changes.

These books often expand on the sensory experiences of caregiving. There have been hints of these in previous chapters, particularly emotional experiences in the work from colonial America, but much of this has been left to our historical imagination. Now we will have some knowledge of the emotional experiences of both ageing and of caregiving. These add considerably to the carerscape, providing personal individual information on the ageing and caregiving relationship, an invaluable aspect which personalises the experiences. So the status and role of carers is becoming increasingly visible.

Mike Hepworth in his introduction to *Stories of Ageing (2000)*says, 'My main aim in writing this book is to encourage you as readers to

B. Hale, *Historical Reflections on Care in the Western World*,
https://doi.org/10.1007/978-3-031-87128-3_10

explore fiction as ageing and care represented in fiction and non-fiction can provide an imaginative resource for understanding variations in the meaning of the experience of ageing in society.' He's right: there is a breadth and depth of personal emotional experiences that can rarely be achieved from a literary ethnographic search.

Stories will expand and substantiate the emotions and inter-relationships of caregiving. They put into the context of everyday life the experiences, emotions, and the morality and spirituality of caregiving, the legalities, and the significance of reciprocity.

This brings me to a more exact description of the sources in this chapter. Those I use here are a small selection from non-fiction and fiction, chosen to represent aspects of caregiving in the nineteenth and twentieth century, through both children's and adult fiction, magazines, movies, and perhaps paintings, though these are more inferential than the other components of the chapter.

Autobiography/biography and novels illustrate personal as well as social/cultural feelings, while children's stories could be said again to show feelings, and to moralise over duty, respect, and reciprocity—providing care to the elderly because care had been provided for the child. And stories for children show details of the problems, what can happen, how it happens, and what is needed to help. They familiarise chronic illness and disability and ageing, by making these visible and by providing explicit processes of understanding and engagement.

Another genre of literature is 'consolation literature' where popular culture encouraged nineteenth-century women to view themselves as a sisterhood of those who bear the 'mark of pain', the mark conferred by caregiving and the experience of the pain of others. Though much of such literature focuses on dying and death, there is also a place for those who are suffering major health problems and those who are caring for them. Diaries and letters often avoid the practical details of physical care to focus on the physical suffering and anguish and their own emotional responses. Magazine articles, as well as books focused on particular topics, can be absorbed into this category.

Yet another interesting field is that of women's magazines, representing both general feelings of experience and also that of moral teaching.

Abel (2000) continues her discussion of what womanhood was about, the definition of female virtue as seen in women's influential literature. Women were encouraged/forced into caregiving with the plethora of women's magazines exhorting that caregiving was a woman's duty, because women are 'calmer, purer, more loving and sensitive than men'. This form of giving is part of womanhood. 'As a dutiful daughter,.... I simply did my job.'

As well as books and magazines, other means of sharing the caregiving experience are now radio, television perhaps and undoubtedly the internet. Media can also include painting and sculpture such as the Roman picture of a woman feeding her imprisoned and sick father from her breasts. Michelangelo's famous sculpture, the Pieta of Mary and Christ in St Peter's evokes tremendous emotion, as do other paintings of this nature. Searching the galleries for pictures of care of the elderly brings forth very little, but portraits of older people themselves are well worth looking at, to see how age is depicted.

Ageing: Adults and Care

Adult fiction is another story, so to speak, and this section will be only a soupcon of favourites. The outstanding care story in my view is *King Lear* and his mixture of un-caring and caring daughters. What a fascinating set of family relationships to study and disentangle, and how far did they help the old man? King Lear with his three daughters, Goneril, Regan, and Cordelia, the one who did care for him as he lost his wits. Duty and affection is expressed in her returning from banishment to take care of her witless father. Was this a sign of old age disabilities, maybe such as Alzheimer's? Did Lear show 'signs of mental deterioration due to old age'. British actor Simon Russell Beale is reported in an AI general discussion saying that medical research he did in preparation to play Lear suggested that the monarch could have been suffering from Lewy Body dementia.

From Shakespeare, I make a leap to Jane Austen whose ageing sounds rather pleasant, although we do know she herself suffered.

'By the bye, as I must leave off being young, I find many Douceurs in being a sort of Chaperon for I am put on a Sofa near the Fire & can drink as much wine as I like,' as Jane says in a letter to Cassandra on 6 November 1813.

While her letters say very little of caregiving, the novels themselves suggest issues. Think of Miss Bates looking after her old mother. What else could she do? And what would happen after Mrs Bates died? Would Miss Bates go on to be a companion aka carer for other people? Or would her niece, Jane Fairfax, care for her despite marrying one of the less heroic men in Austen-land.

Read in Chapter VIII, Vol III about 'old John Abdy's son' who wanted to speak with him. John Abdy was bedridden and very poorly with the rheumatic gout in his joints:

> And poor John's son came to talk to Mr Elton about relief from the Parish: he is very well-to-do himself, you know, being head man at the Crown, ostler and every thing of that sort, but still he cannot keep his father without some help.

And what about Emma and Mr Woodhouse. He needed considerable help in his activities of daily living. Deciding what to send as a gift is only one of the many activities that Emma does to assist her father. She helps him stay oriented, does the conversational work for him, and plays a simple game with him rather than the more complicated ones she prefers.

Think of Emma Woodhouse herself, unwilling to marry because she could not leave her father. She could have left him to servants or her sister. But duty told her to care for him. From a blog by Marilyn Brant comes the information that Jane's ideas for her characters included imagining the lives beyond what she had actually written. One of these was that Mr Woodhouse survived Emma's marriage and kept her and Mr Knightley from settling at Donwell for two years. And Jane Fairfax, delicate Jane Fairfax only lived another nine or ten years after her marriage to Frank Churchill. So would he have had to care for her? It seems likely but from what we know or infer of Frank Churchill, would he really have cared?

Other stories, such as *The Watsons* infer more caregiving. Jane's sister, Cassandra, passed on some detail of The Watsons where she outlined what Jane had intended for the principal character. Mr Watson was to die, then Emma, the principal character, was to become dependent for a home on her narrow-minded sister-in-law and brother. Perhaps she would end up caring for one or other, or even both.

The characters which intrigue me most however are in *Emma* published in 1816, and I return to Miss and Mrs Bates. Was Miss Bates representational of impoverished unmarried women such as family friend Mary Benn, an impoverished spinster of gentle birth but scanty means who was subject to the whims of distant family members, even regarding her domestic circumstances—her home had to be changed several times at the convenience of others. Given exposure to 'old maids' like Mary

Benn and Austen's good friend Anne Sharp—who was also forced into an unsettled life working in different posts as a companion, teacher, and governess throughout her life—one would expect perhaps a more sympathetic portrayal of Miss Bates, whose representation in Emma largely echoes the era's stereotyping of the ageing unmarried woman.

The interesting part of this is that the unmarried women are at the convenience of others, hence their subsequent dependency. Caring done by dependants? It sounds most likely here. What was the cost to those who carried it out? Do we have a division into caring as a burden, and view the impoverished relative as being forced into gratitude and willingness to care for the privilege of being cared for in the sense of given a home and food and place by the hearth? Reciprocity might come at a price.

Temporality is also a big issue in caregiving. Caring there might be in two senses: active, hands-on nursing-type care of the elderly invalid (for want of a better word) and care of the family's impoverished relatives. But what happened before caring was needed? And what happened afterwards? What was the life course of the single woman caregiver then?

Another of our big name samples is Charles Dickens, one of the first people who comes to mind when caring is considered.

Dickens portrays kindly caring: in *Great Expectations*, Dickens describes 'the Aged P' as 'A very old man in a flannel coat; clean, cheerful, comfortable and well cared for, but intensely deaf' and also to more fanciful—'The Aged might have passed for some clean old chief of a savage tribe, just oiled.' He's also described as having 'quite a rakish air'.

Such an elderly man 'required as much watching as a powder mill,' says Dickens, no doubt because of the Aged P's liking to read the newspaper aloud by the light of candles, as Wemmick tells Pip.

Interestingly, when Pip is brought low by the machinations of Miss Havisham (an evil old lady), Wemmick tells him that it would do him good 'to have a perfectly quiet day with the Aged'. Pip adds: 'I soon fell asleep before Wemmick's fire, and the Aged and I enjoyed one another's society by falling asleep before it more or less all day.'

Sentimental, doubtless, but the Aged P is a fine vision of old age contentment. He can't hear the tittle-tattle and nonsense of the world and is happy enough with his lot if someone just toasts him a sausage at the fireplace. Sounds good to me.

But there's much more to caring than that gentle companionship. The list is lengthy; thank you to friend Nick Clark who has itemized informally here his Dickens knowledge for this chapter:

> Mary Graham does her part in caring for old Martin Chuzzlewit. She's not his daughter but is a ward. Agnes Wickfield attempts to care for her father when he's under the tyrannical grasp of Uriah Heep. Annie Strong also shows care for Dr Strong, her much older husband (CD leads us to believe that for some of the novel she dallies with the reprobate Jack Maldon). In the same novel Mrs Steerforth requires the help of her companion Rosa Dartle; it's a truly love hate relationship. Judy is also tasked with helping to look after her awful Grandfather Smallweed in Bleak House. The aged Mrs Skewton also requires care in Dombey and Son. Florence also returns to look after her father when his empire collapses, his wife runs off and he feels himself totally alone. Florence also looks after the dying little Paul Dombey. Lucie Mannette takes care of her father Dr Mannette on his release from the Bastille in A Tale of Two Cities. Amy Dorrit cares for her father both when he is imprisoned in the Marshalsea and as he wanders toward death on his 'freedom'. I don't know if he really falls all that correctly into this category but there's also Philip Swidger from (appropriately) the fifth and final Christmas Book The Haunted Man, who is fondly regarded by his son William. Philip is in relatively good shape although he makes quite a thing of telling everyone that he's eighty-seven years of age.

We might consider, too, the circumstances of the brave and resolute Betty Higden from Our Mutual Friend, a staunchly proud but poor, elderly woman who would rather suffer death than face the indignity of the Poor House.

Think too of Dickens himself. He took responsibility for his parents when they go older. His father, John, a problem when Charles was younger, continued to borrow money, using Dickens's name. But Dickens continued to support him, even writing about an operation which his father had to endure. And at the same time Dickens wrote about his mother's dementia. Care in Dickens' terms ranges from companionship to mockery. As an ideology, Victorian domesticity pivots on two figures: the figure of separate spheres and the figure of the domestic woman. The binary logic of separate spheres identifies a private domain where femininity, leisure, feeling, and an ethic of care coalesce in opposition to a public domain where masculinity, work, industry, endurance, and an ethic of achievement preside.[1] So says Monica F. Cohen who portrays the figure of the middle-class domestic woman, with household managerial skills joined to an ethic of care. Thus was the home idealized.

What comes from these nineteenth-century stories? Duty, companionship, emotions, support, help of various sorts when required, self-righteousness, and self-gratification.

Onwards from the nineteenth to the twentieth century—and let's not forget that these beginning stories are selections and there are many more books and stories out there to be read.

Still Alice

So first of all, try this novel then film adaptation of forgetfulness and the spiral of Alzheimer's, *Still Alice* by Lisa Genova, neuroscientist and author.

Alice Howland is proud of the life she has worked so hard to build. A Harvard professor, she has a successful husband and three grown children. When Alice begins to grow forgetful at first she just dismisses it, but when she gets lost in her own neighbourhood she realizes that something is terribly wrong. Alice finds herself in the rapid downward spiral of Alzheimer's disease. She is only 50 years old. This incredibly moving story was filmed with Julianne Moore who won the, movie released in 2014, Best Actress Academy Award for her performance.

For caregivers? Read how the husband reacts to his wife's diagnosis, and how the children struggle. Caregiving is an emotional change of role, perceptions of the person and relationships.

Read more of Lisa Genova's work—not necessarily fitting in with the care of the elderly, but certainly bringing alive the experiences of caregivers. And also, reminding us that there's another person in this experience, the 'caree' or cared-for. What's it like to be looked after, cared for all the time? To be losing abilities?

Consider this: *No Saints Around Here: A Caregiver's Days*. Here we have a non-fiction account by Susan Allen Toth, with the description in the blurb, as follows:

'Wrenching, occasionally peevish, at times darkly funny, and always deeply felt, Toth's intimate, unsparing account reflects the realities of seeing a loved one out of life: 'the critical support of some friends and the disappearance of others; the elasticity of time, infinitely slow and yet in such short supply; the sheer physicality of James's decline and the author's own loneliness; the practical challenges—the right food, the right wheelchair, the right hospital bed—all intricately interlocking parts of the act of loving and caring for someone who in so many ways is fading away.'

Pick out the caregiving issues here: the practicalities of caregiving intertwined with the emotions of watching a loved one slowly die; the consequent sadness and grieving; closer friendships or a fading of friends and subsequent isolation; temporality of the caregiving, the illness and the time left to live; the physical and emotional tiredness.

For the caregiver's responses, Walter Mosley's novel, *The Last Days of Ptolemy Grey* describes the reaction of non-kin who becomes a caregiver. The synopsis reads: 'Ptolemy Grey is a 91 year old man who is marooned in his apartment that is overflowed with moments from the past'. This fictional tale deals with the unexpected twists and turns that come at the end of people's lives.

And caring? Ptolemy is too suspicious of anyone else to allow them into his life, until he meets Robyn, his niece's seventeen-year-old lodger at his grandnephew's funeral, and the only one willing to take care of an old man.

But Robyn will not tolerate Ptolemy's hermit-like existence. She challenges him to interact more with the world around him, and he grasps more firmly onto his disappearing consciousness. Mosley makes you understand the problems by his description of moving

'He tried to get to his feet by leaning forward and pushing on the arms of the chair. He failed first and second times. He made it on the third. Standing up hurt in three places: his elbow, his knee and ankle.'

That's something of what it's like to be an ageing, disabled person—difficulty moving, and pain. And in need of care.

And we have Ethan Frome, from Edith Wharton, one of the first unsentimental depictions in American literature of the impact of illness and trauma on a family. Many people are nostalgic about a past where families took care of their own without outside help or complaint. This romanticized past is put to rights in Wharton's description of desolation, with the bleak poverty and isolating winters in rural late nineteenth-century New England. Somebody had to stay and care for the folks. 'There warn't ever anybody but Ethan. Fust his father…then his mother…then his wife.'

Next I want to put forward *Tuesdays with Morrie* by Mitch Alborn which less of an actual hands-on caregiving but more in the nature of a close relationship, companionship situation, when a former student visits his old professor every Tuesday (hence the title), and the story progresses from former learning to learning how to live, and obviously how to be with someone dying.

Then *Scar Tissue* by Michael Ignatieff, deals with dementia, following a family through the tensions and upheavals after a mother's diagnosis. Similarly, Sally Magnusson's, *When the Memories Go* is a moving account of remembering the good days while dealing with the onset and continuation of dementia. Her analysis of the disease and her investigation into care is not only part of 'consolation' literature, but part of our learning about what dementia is, how we all differ in our dealings with it and what it means to us, both personally and as a society.

And for a final tip, read the novel *One True Thing* by Anna Quindlen, a contemporary novel which deals with the gender expectation of women who will care, while men continue on their own paths. Ellen Gulden's father hints that she must leave her successful job as a New York journalist to come home and care for her cancer-sick mother. The phrase 'what about my life?' has a poignancy which all caregivers can relate to. And during the caregiving time, the relationship of the two women changes and deepens.

Back to Australia where Henry Handel Richardson's focus on Richard Mahony's problems is accompanied by vivid descriptions of the effect on his caregiving wife.

And there are more such books where the caregiver is a major protagonist.

Movies

As for movies, dementia seems to be the keynote for films. The first I remember was *Iris*, based on her husband and caregiver's memories of Iris Murdoch's development of dementia.

Based on the book *Elegy for Iris* by John Bayley, this movie tells the true story of English novelist Iris Murdoch's descent into Alzheimer's disease and the unconditional love of Bayley, her partner of 40 years.

As well as *Still Alice*, we also have *Alice Cares*, a documentary on robots helping as companions and assistants to older people living alone because of the increasing population. The World Health Organization says that the number of 80 year olds is expected to triple between 2020 and 2050 to reach 426 million. Of these, many will need some sort of in-home health care; others might become lonely and could develop dementia. *Alice Cares*, a fascinating documentary from Dutch Sander Burger, examines a pilot programme developed by researchers at Amsterdam's Free University that is testing the use of an emotionally intelligent 'care-bot' named Alice with the elderly population. A remarkable representation of how technology can be combined with human care to support seniors living independently, this fest favourite should wind up on the radar of cable programmers and academics.

Manufactured by the US firm, Hanson Robotics, Alice is approximately 2 feet tall, with a soft, doll-like face and a camera behind her blinking eyes. As someone from the research group explains, 'People are afraid of big robots.' The software that drives her combines results from lab experiments, field studies, focus groups and computer simulations. Perhaps the most exciting part of the pic is the opportunity to see Alice at work. Burger follows the development of the relationship between Alice and each of the three widowed seniors— Martha Remkes, Carolien Schellekens-Blanke, and Jo Van Wittmarschen— to whose apartments she is brought on a regular basis by the research team. Although all the women initially maintain that they would prefer to have a real person coming in, Alice is able to engage each of them in conversation and relate to them in different ways. She watches TV soccer matches with Remkes (who dresses her in team colours), even exclaiming, "Go Holland go" to wake her when she dozes off; she sings and plays music with Schellekens-Blanke, a vocalist; and she monitors and counts out Van Wittmarschen's physical therapy exercises.

Another movie, *The Savages*, is about Jon and Wendy Savage, two siblings who have spent their adult years trying to recover from their abusive father, Lenny. Suddenly, a call comes in that Lenny's girlfriend has died and he cannot care for himself. Lenny suffers from dementia and her family dumps Lenny on his children. Despite the fact Jon and Wendy have not spoken to Lenny for twenty years and he is even more loathsome than ever, the Savage siblings feel obliged to take care of him. Now together, brother and sister must come to terms with the new and painful responsibilities with their father. The siblings are forced to face the struggle with their own personal demons.

And the Canadian *Still Mine* written and directed by Michael McGowan and based on a true story,[4] the film stars James Cromwell as Craig Morrison, a farmer in rural St. Martins, New Brunswick who battles a government bureaucrat (Jonathan Potts) for the right to build a new house for his ailing wife Irene (Geneviève Bujold) when their existing home no longer suits her health needs

Driving Miss Daisy is a goodie, with an elderly woman developing a heartwarming relationship with the driver whose she needs to her get around.

More caregiver books, some fiction, some 'how to' books can be found on the internet, needless to say, on https://www.homehelpershomecare.com/blog/2015/08/caregiver-books.

Themes? Conclusions?

What do we have, what can we learn from the list of stories? Is there a major theme in caring literature? Arthur Kleinman introduces limbo, the liminal, the in-between, a significant anthropological concept:

> The chronically ill often 'are like those trapped at a frontier, wandering confused in a poorly known border area, waiting desperately to return to their native land....This image should also alert us to the...entrance and exit formalities...and especially [to] the relatives and friends who press their faces against windows to wave a sad goodbye, who carry sometimes the heaviest baggage, who sit in the same waiting rooms, and who even travel through the same land of limbo, experiencing similar worry, hurt, uncertainty and loss.... (p. 183)

And isn't this the same for caregivers and caregiving? This is the main reason for us to identify and emphasize the role—to make the process visible, to alleviate the isolation, the loneliness and the confusion, and to offer a sense of belonging with others in the same situation.

Carol Levine (2014) says that 'In an aging society, when medical miracles save and prolong lives but do not necessarily cure, caregiving is becoming a normative experience.' A quick survey of the internet will support her comments. Caregiving, from being invisible, is now a most thoroughly researched topic in health and in the social sciences.

She also says in her various works that most caregivers are family members, who feel isolated and confined, and aware that there is a difficult journey ahead, undertaken out of love or obligation. But as Levine remarks, there are no systems to guide these caregivers.

> [...] isolated, confined and unsure of when or where or how the difficult journey will end! It is a journey that most embark on out of love or obligation. And yet there are no maps or GPS systems to guide confused travellers.

She has produced the most articulate and moving set of 'story behind the stories' that we could find. The insights of the stories she has selected can act as the guides or maps to caregivers, and importantly too, to those of us who try to help, support, and guide/inform caregivers. Not only does she provide a stellar set of stories on caregiving, but also includes further references.

When Carol was writing, there may have been few route maps to caregiving. Now the bookshops and the internet abound with numerous books on how to care, caring for yourself as the caregiver, finding help, emotional concerns, and other related topics. Maps there are now in plenty. Nell Casey has edited a collection of memoirs by well-known writers whose autobiographical and fictional stories provide warning signs in plenty, and who place caregiving in its liminal position as an in-between role in the case of a child caring for a parent, the role is unclear. It is neither a child nor a parent, for example, without a parent to care for, orphan, without a parent, experienced adult, resumption of a usual life, whatever that might be. Lioness Ayres writes about our stories of caregiving: stories of ideal lives, of ordinary lives, of compromised lives, and ambiguous stories. She suggests that her findings demonstrate diverse meanings which caregivers make of their lives.

Read, mark, and digest!

And, as a hallmark of the role for many, could we consider Auden, in his poem *The More Loving One*. 'Let the loving one be me.'

Recently I found *Communities of Care* by Talia Schaffer, and I'm finding it a splendid read. The focus is on care in Victorian fiction and in the informative blurb, 'In the Victorian era, medical science offered little hope for cure of illness or disability, and chronic invalidism and lengthy convalescences were common. Small communities might gather around afflicted individuals to minister to their needs and palliate their suffering. *Communities of Care* examines these groups in the novels of Jane Austen, Charlotte Brontë, Charles Dickens, George Eliot, Henry James, and Charlotte Yonge, and studies the relationships that they exemplify. '

On page 1, Schaffer quotes Florence Nightingale, '...almost every woman in England has, at one time in her life, [been in] charge of the personal health of somebody,...'.

From there Schaffer looks at Austen, Dickens, and Bronte with aim of developing 'care as a lens through which to view relationships.' (p. 2). Her aim is to develop the category of 'communities of care', a phrase and a lens to enhance our ability to see the issues. Her Introduction is a goldmine of thoughts and ideas.

Conclusion

I began the chapter by suggesting that fiction, non-fiction, and movies might provide us with emotional information on caregiving, as well as the relational information which is so important.

Included in this relational description, we could use the phrase 'emotional labor' defining interactions of care type of work. In this chapter, we can see just what emotional labour can mean. First of all, I suggest the emotional labour lies in the interaction with the cared-for person, and also the interactions with other kin who might or might not be helpful. There are the interactions with the paid and probably more objective health professionals, and further, there are the conscious emotional interactions in the movement of women within their local community, the building of networks through often reciprocal help, but always with the basis of support, assistance, and care.

And there's more, much more. Add to the list on ageing: Diana Athill on her own ageing processes, and Mike Hepworth, combining sociological analysis with gerontology and literature, in considering ageing in fiction, by particular authors such as novelists Agatha Christie, Penelope Lively, and Joanna Trollope.

Check Nell Casey's *Unholy Ghost*, a collection of essays on the personal experiences of some sufferers of depression, and also portraying the damage that their despair brings to the life of others (p. 1). Frank McCourt in *Angela's Ashes* on his own and his family's suffering from his father's alcoholism gives an incredibly vivid and moving picture of the impact of a disease on family members.

And TV? Look out for the comedies such as, for example, *One Foot in the Grave*, and various characters in *Dad's Army*.

What I've offered here is only a bite at the cherry—there's far more in the caregiving role for the elderly but I suggest that with the addition of literature, caregiving is now firmly on the map.

References

Ansello, Edward. 1977. Old Age and Literature: An Overview. *Educational Gerontology* (2): 211–218.

Austen, Jane. 1815. *Emma, pub.* UK: John Murray.

Austen, Jane, 1816, *Emma, pub* John Murray, UK

Austen, Jane. 1803. *The Watsons, pub.* Penguin Classics, 2018.

Brant, Marilyn, Blog April 2016 *All Things Austen, Dear Aunt Jane.*

Dickens, Charles. 1861. *Great Expectations, pub.* . Pengun 1998.

Casey, Nell. 2008. *"An Uncertain Inheritance" Writers on Caring for family.* New York: Morrow.

Cohen, Monica F. 2017. *Domesticity and Victorian Literature.* Literary Studies (19th century).

Hepworth, Mike. 2000. *Stories of Aging.* Buckingham: Open University Press.

Kleinman, Arthur. 1988. *The Illness Narratives: Suffering*, 183. New York: Basic Books.

Levine, Carol. 2014. *In the Land of Limbo.* Nashville, Tennessee: Vanderbilt University Press.

McDivitt, Lindsey. https://www.lindseymcdivitt.com/about/

Poirier, Suzanne, and Pioness Ayres. 2002. *Stories of Family Caregiving: Reconsiderations of Theory, Literature and Life.* Indianapolis, IN: Sigma Theta Tau Intl (1 April 2002)

Schaffer, Talia. 2021. *Communities of Care: The Social Ethics of Victorian Fiction.* Princeton, New Jersey: Princeton University Press.

Somerville, H. 1929. *Madness and Shakespeare.* London: Richards Press.

https://www.nytimes.com/2015/12/20/opinion/jane-austens-guide-to-alzheimers.html

https://www.senioradvisor.com/blog/2014/11/movies-for-caregivers-7-films-about-family-friends-love-and-loss/

CHAPTER 11

Identity and Voice

History of any kind tends to sprawl, says Bill Bryson (2011) in his discussion of home and privacy. And he comments that history is about ordinary things. Surely both these observations are true of caregiving. It sprawls over time in a variety of ages, for a number of people, different situations from intimate personal care to a social acknowledgement of disabilities and ageing. And there is a variety of actions and interactions, mostly in one place: at home, living within a community. The question arises: does informal care continue in a different sense if the cared-for individual is admitted to institutional care? Is there an aspect of caregiving of a major emotional component then?

It is a story of the ordinary everyday efforts in living. Much of it is invisible, happening in this place of home, with the role of caregiver emerging, often bit by bit, as needs change. But the extra activities and time taken to care has an impact on the emergent caregiver. So it is special as old skills are used and often new skills learned. Gavin Francis (2015) says in his concluding chapter that all of us have landscapes we consider special: places which are charged with meaning, for which we feel affection or reverence. I suggest that caregiving is such a landscape for many of us, holding the same meanings—affection or anger, power or helplessness, memories and present-day happenings. And we can add to these.

What more can we add? Gender? Either men or women, or trans gender. Does this matter? We need to find out. Payment? Carers'

B. Hale, *Historical Reflections on Care in the Western World*, https://doi.org/10.1007/978-3-031-87128-3_11

allowances in different countries, which mark the value of the work, support the caregiver and, in some cases, save due to the more expensive informal care. And we need to consider employment for caregivers alongside care responsibilities. And how about carer-friendly workplaces? More detail in the next chapter.

So we have a number of features which can construct a caregiving role, and also others which add to the maintenance of older people at home. And we are now in the twenty-first century: the history of caregiving recognition began in the late twentieth century as Timothy Cook (2007) points out.

Everyday situations arise: how noisy is it and is that bearable? How do caregivers touch, what are the emotions in caregiving, and in receiving care? How affectionate should the caregiver be? Is there a possibility of abuse in the relationship—from either side? Too many and harsh demands on the caregiver perhaps, or cruelty from the caregiver to the elderly.

Further than that are other and wider questions: household space, for example, and how much is given up to care, one bed, one room? And is the caregiver linked in with other domestic roles such as childcare, domestic work?

Wider still—how much of care is influenced by spirituality of what should be done, and how much by reciprocity—legally, the giving of goods and money on death of the elderly, and the expectation of the caregiver that when her/his turn comes, someone will do the same as she/has done.

The specific role is to give care, tend, look after, and ensure well-being as far as possible. The influences are both personal, social expectations, and legal and spiritual.

That's the role.

How about individuals' emotions, health, and need for support?

I want to introduce some contemporary caregivers, to meet real people in their current situations. The first belongs to the information I used from our group, to write an article for the local Journal of Social Work (carer names anonymously of course and with permission and some amusement from group members). It indicates caregiving by a spouse as a journey from the 'we' to 'I'.

The others are case studies. To my mind they indicate the importance of sharing our knowledge with each other.

These things are important indeed. But so are the small things, the intimate knowledge, the watchfulness, the care. Such as in the following:

Bob and Eliza

Bob was in hospital, in long-term care.

'Bob isn't hungry, doesn't eat' was the report. 'Doesn't he like the food?' the group asked.

'He'll eat if I feed him, but I can't be here at every mealtime…I do try.'

The group murmured agreement. Eliza went on, 'When I come in, I pick up his sandwiches from the end of the bedtable and unwrap them for him.'

Pause for thought. Nellie in the group asked,

'At the end of the table?'

'That's right. He's not interested, the staff say, he could reach out for them, and he can unwrap them, take off the covering, but doesn't want to.'

Nellie said, 'Can he see them?' Someone else said, 'My Bill used to be like that until I put the food right under his nose.'

Chuckles from the women, murmurs of 'that's men for you, dish it up right in front of them.' But Eliza was faraway.

'I wonder….I wonder if he does see them…if he can stretch out…he doesn't turn much, doesn't turn his head….'

Upshot? Put the sandwiches in front of Bob, he could then see them. He could bend his head and look. And yes, he could unwrap them. Unwieldy, clumsy, and slow—but he could do it!

The space of what we can see, turn to look, hear. A caregiver has to be fully aware of the implications of the needs.

And the next story tells us of an emotional dilemma.

Bill and Cathy

At home. Bill is noisy at night. Cathy can't sleep. He's restless, sighing, grunting, groaning, snoring. Moves when he can.

'What will I do? I want a good night's sleep!' Cathy brought the problem to the group.

As usual, Nellie was one of the first to answer.

'Got a spare room?'

'Yes, a couple, used to be the kids' rooms.'

'Move into one of them?'

'But we've never been apart, not in 55 years!'

'There's always a first time.'

Someone else asked: 'Does he need help at night?'

'No…he's just noisy, got a catheter so doesn't have to get up to pee.'

'Then if you want a good night's sleep, you move, girl!'

Cathy did, and cried herself to sleep, as she reported, for the first few nights, and maybe longer.

Then!

Bill moved into care.

'You could move back into your own bedroom, now.' Nellie told her.

'Can't. He might come home. And ..'

Eventually we got from her that she didn't want to be in the bedroom she'd shared with her husband. If he had to be in what she called 'a strange bed', she would be in 'a strange bed' too. Only when Bill died did she feel she could move back.

The psychology of this defeated our pundits in the group. But she was happy. She felt she had shown caring by moving as he had done, into a separate room.

There are more stories, as many stories as there are caregivers.

But now to look for help for carers. How do you get it?

Informal help there is in plenty. As we said in our *Family Care* book (Barrett et al. 2013), there is social capital out there. Social capital there was in plenty for Chrissy to draw on, living in a small town as she had done for years. She hung out sheets day after day—and the neighbours came round to ask what was up, how was she, and could they help?

This is community care—just as it was in early America, just as it was in mediaeval and Renaissance times, and in early Christian times, and probably in earlier times too. The type of help may differ in detail, but the goodwill is there.

Other stories? Aplenty!

Nellie in tears. 'He won't let me see the grandchildren'… We worked out a solution to that one. Fast! And Nellie got to see her grandchildren.

Alice's husband wouldn't let anyone else do anything for him. She had to rush into the meeting, keep an eye on the clock, and rush back again. Members of the group took it in turns to get to know her husband and sit with him for a short time so she could get out. This gift was despite all they had to do themselves by way of caregiving.

Val and her husband 'burned rubber' day or night when on demand by mother-in-law.

The group taught Lizzie how to write a cheque and how to go to the bank and get cash. Someone from the group went with her. Her husband had always done it, and she was at a loss when he suffered a stroke.

So the timing of things—as well as the space, as well as relationships—is important as is, of course, the personal knowledge and the slowly acquired knowledge of care for oneself.

The group provided a marvellous outlet where women could sit and talk out their hurts, their anxieties and anger. We encouraged everyone to let it all out.

Professionals at the hospital were exceedingly helpful. The circles of care were in place, from allied health professionals to consultants. Most of the time.

One unforgettable story is that of 'She'll manage.' Said by a new consultant as he discussed the needs and management of a badly depressed man. The wife came stumbling in on a stick, crippled with arthritis. 'She'll manage.'

'How?'

He had no answer. But the carers' group did.

Further up to date information on caregiving takes us from the personal to the somewhat impersonal.

The BBC reports emerging technology that will help distant relatives keep an eye on their elderly or vulnerable people living alone. They do this by monitoring their electricity usage—but as with all innovations, there is the potential for misuse (BBC 23 May 2021, William Kremer reporter).

And taken from the internet is the following information.

CareFlick is a mobile app powered by an AI assistant named Yana that provides personalized support and companionship for caregivers of people with special needs. Key features: AI assistant Yana provides empathetic conversations and support. And suggests personalized activities, therapies and content. 28 Mar 2024.

And yet again, there's more: AI companionship for elderly, AI assistance for people with dementia—the list goes on.

But yes, there are problems. For example, carer leave, employment recognition of carers, the carers' allowance, support for carers, grants—call it what you will—but the recognition of the economic hardships of carers has been acknowledge in the form of recognition and of monetary payments. But there have recently been difficulties with these such as, among others, over-payments, and funding problems.

We need to keep these in mind as we continue creating our carerscape.

References

Barrett, Patrick, Beatrice Hale, and Mary Butler. 2013. *Family Care and Social Capital: Transitions in Informal Care*. London: Springer.

Bryson, Bill. 2011. *At Home: A Short History of Private Life*. New York: Knopf.

Cook, Timothy. 2007. *The History of the Carers' Movement*. London: Carers UK.

Francis, Gavin. 2015. *Adventures in Human Being*. London: Profile Books. Publication in Association with Welcome Collection, London.

Hale, Beatrice, (2000), From Partner to Carer, *Aotearoa NZ Social Work Journal,* Iss.12, pp.7–10.

Hale, Beatrice. 2000. Grassroots Experience. *Aotearoa NZ Social Work Journal*.

CHAPTER 12

Modern Times

To conclude, I want to outline some of the numerous effective caring organisations which have appeared recently, showing the visibility of carers, and the recognition and value of the role. And not only these but also the political resolutions on behalf of caregivers, recognising the role in economic terms. And I refer to Kate Hamblin et al. (2024) for their work on the policies of nine different countries recognising caregiving. As the blurb says,

> Written and informed by national experts, this is the first publication to provide a detailed examination of the development and implementation of carer leave policies and policies in 9 countries across Asia, Oceania, Europe and North America.
> It compares the origins, content and implications of national policies and practices intended to enable workers to provide care to family members and friends while remaining in paid employment—known as 'carer leave'.
> Well worth reading!

The Start

In the United Kingdom in 1954, Mary Webster gave up her work as a congregational minister to care for her parents. She was 31.

In this decade, says Carers UK, she began to think about the problems which this decision had created—financial, in particular. And in 1963,

B. Hale, *Historical Reflections on Care in the Western World*,
https://doi.org/10.1007/978-3-031-87128-3_12

she 'burst upon the public' publicising the major practical difficulties, including financial hardship and isolation that women carers were experiencing. In 1965 she formed the National Council for Single Woman and her Dependants. And she won a battle for a Dependent Relative Tax Allowance in 1967.

From then on her legacy has spawned numerous such national groups.

In 1963, Jill Pitkeathley combined two organisations: National Council for Carers and their Elderly Dependents (previously the NCSWD) with the Association of Carers to create a single voice for carers in the form of the Carers National Association.

This was groundbreaking and ground shaking. Up until then, caregiving had been seen as part of the woman's role, part of the domestic scene, and basically, hidden in a social backroom, if there was such a thing, so that it was simply considered to be something that women did.

Until Mary Webster had made caregiving more visible, and had publicly chronicled the dimensions of the work which caring entailed, caregiving had disappeared into the domestic role. And let's note that we are dealing here with caregiving for different ages, different disabilities, mental and physical; we are not dealing only with the elderly, though that is the focus of this book. In 1981, a new organisation, the Association of Carers, was set up by Judith Oliver, herself a carer of a disabled husband and looking after a young family. Her view was that all carers required support, not just those who had elderly dependants. Thank you to Carers UK and to Tim Cooke for the historical information.

Caregiving—invisible, hidden, unnoticed. Or time-consuming, tiring and knowledgeable. Emotional and relational. We have these in the carerscape and we can throw as many adjectives as we like at the role. They will serve to enhance and emphasize the context of caregiving.

And there is much more on the growth of carer organizations in different countries. We can look at Colombia, Sweden, Canada, Ireland, New Zealand, Australia, Taiwan, and the United States—among others. The list of carer organizations is growing.

Not only that but some organizations are interested in how care has developed in their area, and I discovered work on early Sweden where Birgitta Oden and her colleagues (1995) offer information on the development of care in Sweden and identify similar evidence of caring to what I have found in other parts of Europe and the UK. Six different historical periods are distinguished: early and mediaeval, feudal and Catholic, The Reformation, transition, the liberal and philanthropic period and the welfare state period. This particular work identifies a period of reformation (1550–1700) where new 'Mosaic' laws from central government were imposed. These said that abusive parents (whether physically or verbally) would carry a penalty of capital punishments. At the same time weak persons who were not family members were still cared for within the family. The next period saw the 'disbandment of the religious influence on elderly care'. But at the same time, the first laws about organising public care for weak persons in society were formulated during this period, and gerontologist Birgitta Oden (ibid)wrote that during this period the nuclear family became the ideal in society, and care of old people became the responsibility of the local parish.

Further on, from mid-1800s to the 1930s is what is designated as the liberal and philanthropic period in Sweden.

But back to other countries, and on to the later twentieth century, we have Carers Canada and the Canadian Caregiver Coalition (CCC) forming in 1999 with the original purpose of uniting caregivers, service providers, policy makers and other stakeholders, with a focus on the needs of caregivers.

Initially, members included researchers, government officials, professionals, and organizations with interest in and commitment to caregivers. Through a secretariat, they supported and encouraged research and education activities, undertaking policy work as time and resources permitted. Funding from Pfizer Canada covered CCC's development costs over the first five years of its operation. The J.W. McConnell Family Foundation also contributed funding in support of specific activities.

As well as Carers UK and Carers Canada, there are numerous other national organisations and timewise, the first sections focus on the turn of the century, from the 1990s to the early 2000s. Later sections will take us further.

To begin with, then, for example, we have Carers New Zealand, Carers Australia, and of course carers organisations in the United States, all of whom had the same background and focus—the visibility of caregivers, and identifying and responding to their needs.

In Ireland, the Carers Association was founded in 1987, and in 2006, the Irish census showed a total of 160,917 people who claimed carer status and providing 43 or more hours of care each week. The Association has estimated that carers provide 194 million hours of care a year at a saving of about 2.5 billion euros to the Irish economy. And in further statistics, 33,000 full-time carers qualify for the Carers Allowance from the government.

Taiwan has an Association of Family Caregivers. In 1996, it was the first non-profit organization to voice the rights for family caregivers in Taiwan. The association encourages each city to set up a chapter in order to provide family caregivers with services. The main association is in Taipei and there are ten chapters around Taiwan. The TAFC claims that: (1) the government should share the burden of family carers; (2) the government should provide well-qualified respite services; (3) the government should provide family carers with training and support; (4) labour policy should help employees fulfil their responsibilities as family caregivers.[32]

The TAFC provides family caregivers with a consulting hotline, newsletters of the association, in-service courses for professional personnel, support groups, and counselling services for caregivers. The association has allied with the Welfare Organization of the Elderly, 'Federation for the Welfare of Taiwan's Seniors' https://www.oldpeople.org.tw/pop/pages/55838c705a2941d1b05e7beb08abdf14 Taiwan Long-term Care Professional Association, and Taiwan Alzheimer's Disease Association to build a support network for family caregivers.

There have been numerous surveys, and in the United States one survey in November 2007 showed that most family caregivers felt more positive about their experiences than they did just before they took on the responsibility, with significant differences in expectation prior to becoming a caregiver and the actual experience. This survey also found that caregivers are often burdened by high out-of-pocket costs in caring for a spouse or parent, but from the Utah Parents Center discussion, inclusive of all ages, they say in their Caregiver e-journal:

> Sixty percent of the caregivers called the experience "very or extremely rewarding," a 50% jump over the number of caregivers who thought in advance they would find the experience "very or extremely rewarding." Nearly 80% (78.8%) percent of the caregivers found the experience to be at least "rewarding," an increase of more than one-third from initial expectation. A majority of the caregivers—nearly 54%—formed a stronger bond with the patient during the time they were together.
>
> Almost 60% of the respondents reported an improvement in the quality of their relationship with the person for whom they cared. By contrast, fewer than 10% said that their relationship got worse during the time they were caregivers.

Social activities of the caregiver tend to diminish. The diminished social activities are replaced with an increased quality of relationship with the care recipient.
More than 2/3 of all caregivers (68.7%) said they enjoy the tasks associated with caregiving. Prior to assuming the role, fewer than half (45.5%) thought they would enjoy caregiving.

Further information for the visibility of the role is the amount of research now being carried out on caregiving. A look at the internet will show a considerable number of publications on caregiving.

One of the many worth reading is that of an earlier Caregiver statistics fact sheet (2012) whose content says that 43.5 million of adult family caregivers care for someone 50 + years of age and 14.9 million care for someone who has Alzheimer's disease or other dementia [Alzheimer's Association, 2011/ 2].

And additional information is on the increase of male caregivers, some of whom we have already identified in the earlier centuries as givers of medicine and as writers to medical men on behalf of those illiterates who needed help, of their interest in the care required by their kin, and even to undertaking some hands-on assistance such as observing and perhaps even assisting at times.

The number of male caregivers may be increasing and will continue to do so due to a variety of social demographic factor according to Betty Kramer (1997), and Thompson (2002). Other information about US caregivers: by 2009, more than 61.6 million people provided unpaid care for a chronically ill, disabled or aged family member or friend at an estimated value of $450 billion.

And of further interest, we read that 1.4 million children aged from 8 to 18 provide care for an adult relative; 72% are caring for a parent or grandparent, although most are not the sole caregiver,

30% of family caregivers caring for older individuals are themselves aged 65 or over; another 15% are between the ages of 45 and 54.[23]

Licensing and certification for caregiving can vary by state. In some states, the only licensing needed is by the company that employs the caregivers (unless it is from the state). In other states, an online certification course is recommended. Some states require in-classroom certification, and others require personal care licensing, which can be applied for online. Along with that, in some states, further certifications are required such as CPR training and first aid training.[24]

Some US states, such as California, have set out the responsibilities of the primary caregiver, from the Primary Caregiver Responsibilities, California Dept of Public Health.

Colombia

Although elder care is not the focus in this Colombian initiative, reported in *The Guardian*, 31 May 2024, this is well worth sharing, showing the acknowledgement of the role, and the value of the caregivers.

> In Colombia, like most societies, unpaid caregiving falls disproportionately on women. Few choose to dedicate their life to caring for the young, the old or the sick and most carers have no training, financial assistance or recognition. In 2010 Colombia became the first country in the world to introduce a law that requires the contributions of the invisible care economy to be documented.
>
> When Bogotá's local government studied unpaid care workers in 2018 they found around one in three women in the city—about 1.5 million people—were labouring with little recognition for their dedication, 90% of them living in poverty. Most had no formal education, one in five had a diagnosed illness and 14% were housebound because of the needs of those they care for.
>
> In response, Bogotá's first female mayor, Claudia López, proposed an innovative programme which then beat 630 other applicants to win the Mayors Challenge prize, securing $1m in funding from Bloomberg Philanthropies in January 2022. One of those coordinating the project is Sandra Milena Blanco:
>
> "Most of the time carers have little support or do not know how to access it, which sadly means they have a lot of mental health issues, due to the massive burden they carry," she says. "Sometimes they have to care for two or three people alone and it is not uncommon that the carers themselves are old and need help, they are just too busy caring for others."
>
> The plan involves 23 care blocks strategically dotted around Bogotá's deprived neighbourhoods. Carers can stop by to chat to a therapist, receive legal advice from a lawyer around government support, join workshops or yoga classes, swim, learn computer skills, or just drop off dirty washing. They can also bring the people they care for to get some respite.
>
> "There is a strong focus on gender so that these women feel heard and valued," says Claudia Mirta Luna, who oversees implementation. "It's not just about reducing the load on them but making sure they realise the

importance of their work, they value themselves and realise that 'I can care for others but while still caring for myself.'"
The mayor's office sends specialists into homes, once a week for 12 weeks, to tailor strategies for carers.
Espejo's support has brought confidence and a new contentment to Adriana and to her grandmother. Taylor, Luke (2024) A sense of optimism and the chance to chat: how Bogota is giving respect to unpaid carers, The Guardian, Friday, 31st May. writes of a Colombian situation: 'For the first time in two decades, Rubiano has regular time to herself, to go out, do housework, or just watch television.
In the nine weeks Espejo has been visiting she has taught Adriana to make the bed, dust, wash clothes and prepare food.
"It makes a massive difference," Rubiano says. "I honestly never thought that all of this was possible."
Mirta says these lasting changes are what make the programme so efficient. Carers may only visit for four hours a week for 12 weeks but the result is a new independence.
Rubiano has used her free time to gain a qualification from Bogotá's National Training Service, formally recognising her care experience as the city authorities certify the skills of its caregivers, giving them respect and a way into the workforce should they want it. Rubiano currently depends on the monthly stipend (equivalent to about £100) from the state to support Adriana's learning disabilities and from renting out her spare room. She would like to do more.
"I think I'd like to work with older people," she says. "They've got good stories and great gossip."'
The new Bogotá administration wants to increase the 23 care blocks to 45 by 2035 and has also introduced mobile care centres. The programme has attracted international attention, with interest from Mexico, Chile, the Dominican Republic and Sierra Leone.
"This is a big, ambitious idea to shift the care economy at urban scale." says James Anderson, head of government innovation at Bloomberg Philanthropies.
"This is the right programme, tackling the right set of challenges, at exactly the right time—and that's why cities everywhere are watching closely," Anderson says in the Karuna News of 2024 "Care blocks may have started in Bogotá but they will inspire and spread far beyond."

Australia

According to the Australian Bureau of Statistics 2001 paper on the health and well-being of carers, they save the Australian Federal Government over $30 billion a year, while according to the same statistics, there are over 300,000 young carers (Carers Australia states that a young carer is any carer under the age of 25[1]) with 1.5 million potential young carers, where potential is defined as a young person who lives in a household where there is at least one person who requires full-time care (is disabled, etc.).[2] In 2015, carers provided around 1.9 billion hours of unpaid care.[3] According to a new study by the University of Queensland, Australian carers are providing $13.2 billion worth of free mental health support to their friends and family members. This 'hidden workforce' is equivalent to 173,000 full-time mental health support workers.

In Australia they also have the Australian National Young Carers Action Team (ANYCAT) whose goal is to advocate on behalf of young carers (being young carers themselves); In most states and territories they have an ANYCAT equivalent team or board. In Queensland, this is called the Young Carers Action Board Queensland (YCABQ).

Italy

When compared to all other countries, Italy has the highest percentage of residents aged 65 and older. The life expectancy for males is 76.7 and 82.9 for females, and it is predicted that by 2050 these numbers will reach 81 and 86 years, for men and women, respectively. In addition, the country is faced with a rapidly growing older population and a shortage of younger individuals. Furthermore, the Minister of Labour and Social Policies of Italy stated that the family plays the most important role in the quality of life of elders, and it is the primary care provider for the older populations; however, the government also provides assistance to the family caregiver by the following services.

"Qualified assistance at home"
"Support services"
"Service vouchers"
"Daytime centres to provide support for families by offering old people rehabilitation and recreation"
"Stays in holiday resorts for non-self-sufficient old people—including those staying in hospitals or homes"

The family plays an important role in providing care to its older parents but many children still have to work so that they can survive financially, and as a result, many caregivers are immigrant workers. These immigrant workers come in search of work from many parts of the world such as Moldavia, the Philippines, and Peru; however, the largest population of immigrant workers come from the Ukraine. Many of the caregivers work long hours and weeks, and also leave their own families behind and send them the money they make.

UK

According to Carers UK, and based on the 2001 Census, around six million people in the UK provide care on an unpaid basis for a relative, friend, or neighbour in need of support due to old age, disability, frailty or illness. The population of carers is dynamic: at least a third of all people will fulfil a caring role at some point in their lives.

Research has shown that becoming a carer can have many impacts on a person's life. These include financial costs, exclusion and discrimination at work, social isolation, and poor health through stress and physical injury.

At least half of all carers are in full or part-time employment and some care for more than one person. Carers save the UK economy an estimated £87bn a year, https://www.scotlandscensus.gov.uk/search-the-census#/[13] and economic considerations form a key element in government policy to support carers.

And not only do we consider older carers but, in the 2001 Censushttps://en.wikipedia.org/wiki/United_Kingdom_Census_2001 it is indicated that there are 175,000 young carers aged under 18 in the UK today. A poll commissioned by The Princess Royal Trust for Carers in 2004 indicates that the number of young carers could be much higher. But overall for caregiving later, the 2021 Census has revealed approximately still 5.8 million people provide unpaid care across the UK, with 4.7 million in England and 310,000 in Wales.

Scotland

Policy and legislation in relation to caregivers living in Scotland is somewhat different from that in England, Wales, and Northern Ireland. https://en.wikipedia.org/wiki/Countries_of_the_United_Kingdom Carers are defined by the Scottish Census as being 'individuals who look after, or give any help or support to family members, friends, neighbours and others because of long-term physical or mental ill health or disability or problems related to old age' (Scotland's Census Results Online [SCROL]). Estimates from the 2001 Census put the numbers of carers in Scotland at 481,579. Of these, 175,969 are reported to provide more than 20 hours of care a week, and 24% provide more than 50 hours of care.

Carers who provide care for 20 hours a week or more are regarded as being at the 'heavy end' of caring (Parker 1990). This assumes that they are the most involved carers, providing both personal and physical care, resulting in high levels of stress and most in need of support services. Many of these carers continue to provide care without support from social work or health services and because of this they remain hidden or invisible (Cavaye 2006; Scottish Executive 2006).

Carers are viewed by the government as an important resource and in recent years have been given increasing recognition in health and social care policy. Since devolution in 1999 legislation and policy for care-givers has been developed by the former Scottish Executive (now Scottish Government).

Carers in Scotland are regarded as 'partners' in the provision of care. As a result, support services provided to carers are regarded as part of the overall package of care to the person being looked after. This means at this time that carers are not seen as service users and are therefore not responsible for the cost of any service provided. The exception to this is when a carer is looking after their partner; in that situation their income may be taken into account during a financial assessment.

This situation was different from that which existed at that time in England where carers were viewed as services users in their own right and as such are liable for the cost of services provided. Yet, in many cases, it is not the carer who actually needs the service; it is the person being cared for who needs it because of their illness or disability. But now Carers Trust Scotland's vision is that unpaid carers are heard and valued as well as freely having access to support, advice and resources to enable carers to live fulfilled lives.

New Zealand

And now, what about the physical and financial aspects? There is now in New Zealand as well as other countries, a carer's allowance. It helps a little.

Prior to 2013, the Ministry of Health did not pay family members as caregivers but several judicial rulings since found this breached the Bill of Rights Act by discriminating against them.

The previous national government then passed legislation allowing some payments but under strict criteria.

In general, we need to be aware that this is only a selection of interesting and intriguing facts, not only emphasizing the carer role, but giving it a robust status, beyond that of the domestic, and underlining the current visibility of carers.

And there's more. A look on the internet will bring you immediate information on carers and the care they themselves are receiving.

International

On 27 February 2004, the International Alliance of Carers Organizations (IACO) was launched by family caregiving organizations from Australia, the UK, Sweden, the Netherlands, and the US. The mission of the organization is threefold:

> [...] to increase visibility of family caregiving across the lifespan as an international issue
> to promote the sharing of best practices in caregiving programmes between countries; and
> to encourage and provide assistance to countries interested in developing family carer organizations.

IACO is headquartered in London. Initial IACO projects included promotion of a United Nations Day for Carers and a presentation on the IACO as part of a half-day workshop at the International Federation on Aging conference in Singapore on 4 August 2004. National family carer organizations in all countries are encouraged to join the alliance.

A look at the Internet shows us the countries within IACO and the number of carers in each country, providing a 'global state of caring'. In addition to IACO, there is also Carers Worldwide. Begun in 2012, this organization exists to care and promote care for the Global South. Based in London, it is remarkably similar in ideals to IACO, and hosts interesting events, including one in 2023 which aimed at empowering unpaid family carers in Nepal to provide health and well-being support to other carers. (see website Carers Worldwide). https://www.carersworldw ide.org.

A look on the internet will provide further information on both these splendid organisations, and will emphasize the importance of unpaid care and highlight its special role.

References

Oden, B., (1995) Interrelations between Generations *in Historical Perspective in Preparation for Aging*, Springer.

Kramer, Betty (1997) Gain in the Caregiving Experience, where are we, what next? *Gerontologist, Apriln 37*(2) 218–32.

And Thompson, Edward H, Jr, (2002), *Men as caregivers: Theory, research and service,* Springer Pub. Company

Index

A

abuse, 6, 14, 39, 51, 52, 72, 79, 80, 109, 117, 126, 140, 141, 153, 176

adopted kin, 49, 70, 73

age/ageing, 1, 4–8, 11, 15, 17, 20, 25–27, 29, 30, 34, 37, 40, 42, 43, 47, 48, 56, 57, 61, 65–70, 72, 73, 76, 77, 80, 85–87, 92, 94, 98, 103–105, 107, 110, 113, 119, 126–129, 135, 136, 140–142, 144, 145, 147, 151–154, 161–163, 165, 166, 168, 173, 175, 185, 188–190

America, 8, 9, 139–141, 145, 152, 154, 161, 178, 181

Appudurai, 5, 8

B

bodies, 43, 50, 93, 126, 134

bodily care, 1, 50, 68, 70, 74, 93, 118, 150

burden, 1, 2, 12, 26, 29, 30, 55, 76, 106, 129, 135, 154, 165, 184, 186

C

Carerscape, 7–9, 12, 14, 22, 23, 57, 61, 80, 120, 147, 161, 179, 182

Carers UK, 181–183, 189

community care, 83, 111, 135, 178

D

diaries, 2, 6, 9, 126, 130, 133, 139, 141, 145, 148, 157, 162

E

economics, 6, 14, 15, 21, 30, 32, 90, 110, 131, 142, 147, 151–153, 158, 179, 181, 189

Egyptian, 3, 38–41, 43, 45, 46, 49, 50, 52–55, 57, 66, 69, 77

ethnoscape, 8

B. Hale, *Historical Reflections on Care in the Western World*,
https://doi.org/10.1007/978-3-031-87128-3

F
fables, 27
fictive kin, 49, 57, 71, 73, 90, 150
folklore, 25–27, 31, 32

G
Greece, 8, 37, 61–65, 69, 77, 79, 80, 83, 140
groups, 2, 5–7, 19, 25, 31, 61, 67, 70, 83, 84, 87, 89, 94–98, 152, 170, 172, 182, 184

H
hands-on care, 46, 75, 98, 106, 150

I
incontinence, 3, 77, 87, 105, 106, 116
Index of Care, 14, 19

L
legal, 5, 37, 39, 48, 51, 55, 70–74, 78, 103, 107, 117, 176, 186
letters, 2, 6, 9, 53, 139, 141, 145, 157, 162, 163

M
mediaeval, 3, 8, 9, 103, 105, 106, 109, 115, 142, 178, 182
movies, 3, 6, 9, 161, 162, 169, 170, 173

N
Neanderthal, 8, 11, 12, 16, 19, 20, 25, 32, 56

O
orthotics, 1, 50, 118, 119

P
paramone, 49
parish(es), 6, 8, 9, 108, 110–113, 117, 121, 127, 131–136, 155, 164, 183
prehistory, 21, 22
productivity, 6, 14, 23, 42, 105, 147
prosthetics, 3, 37, 65, 76, 77, 80, 105, 118, 119

S
Sarah, Gillespie, 147, 148
shabti, 3, 38, 50
slaves, 9, 39, 45, 46, 48, 49, 51, 56, 57, 62, 63, 69–71, 74, 76, 80, 86–88, 90, 92, 134, 139, 144, 152–156, 158
sources, 1, 3–6, 32, 37, 38, 40, 41, 51, 52, 61, 66, 76, 87, 89, 93, 105, 126, 127, 129, 135, 139, 154, 162
space, 4, 8, 45, 52, 67, 76–78, 90–92, 96, 106, 108, 110, 114, 116, 117, 121, 135, 145, 146, 149, 151, 176, 177, 179
spirituality, 2, 4, 8, 9, 41, 54, 57, 61, 72, 78–80, 83, 84, 88, 94, 98, 99, 106, 114, 162, 176

The manufacturer's authorised representative in the EU is Springer Nature Customer Service Centre GmbH, Europaplatz 3, 69115 Heidelberg, Germany. If you have any concerns regarding our products, please contact ProductSafety@springernature.com

Printed and bound by CPI Group (UK) Ltd, Croydon, CR0 4YY
22/09/2026
02220962-0003